T0348794

The Pursuit of Happiness in America

Brian J. Jones

The Pursuit of Happiness in America

A Sociological Perspective

palgrave
macmillan

Brian J. Jones
Villanova University
Villanova, PA, USA

ISBN 978-3-031-65606-4   ISBN 978-3-031-65607-1   (eBook)
https://doi.org/10.1007/978-3-031-65607-1

This Palgrave Macmillan imprint is published by the registered company Springer Nature Switzerland AG.
The registered company address is: Gewerbestrasse 11, 6330 Cham, Switzerland

If disposing of this product, please recycle the paper.

To Suzanne, Megan, Chris, and assorted Joneses: you have made me very happy.

PREFACE

This book has been a long journey to an unintended—but happy—destination.

Around the turn of the century, I took the first step. Alarmed by the rising tide of opinion that American society was in decay, I acted like a sociologist. I built a model of our everyday social lives in work, family, voluntary association, and social networks. After digging a theoretical foundation, I got to work filling the framework with data from the General Social Survey. Thus was constructed *Social Capital in America* (2011).

That book provided a direct look at the social structures we build and maintain in our personal lives (which is why I subtitled it "Buried Treasure"). But over time it became clear that something was missing: how Americans *feel* about their social capital. In 2019 I published *Social Capital in American Life,* which added attitudes such as job satisfaction, family satisfaction, trust, and, yes, happiness to the model. Not surprisingly, the time we invest in everyday social structures often pays off in personal satisfaction.

Happiness is an internet singularity. It powerfully attracts poets, preachers, philosophers, and, especially, psychologists to offer commentary. In a way, the central project of sociology is to reveal the significance of the social structures all around us. One of those revelations is how powerfully they resonate within. As you are about to read, happiness is a sociological reality.

Havertown, PA   Brian J. Jones

CONTENTS

LIST OF FIGURES

LIST OF TABLES

CHAPTER 1

On Happiness

Abstract Every discipline and every person seeks the keys to happiness. Sociology searches for them by focusing on its central concept, social structure. That search is facilitated in this volume by five decades of the General Social Survey, the gold standard for quantitative research. It is complemented by qualitative questions administered by a professional interviewing firm asking for people's personal insights into happiness.

Keywords Happiness • General Social Survey • Qualitative interviews

> The purpose of life is to find happiness.
> - the Dalai Lama

Happiness advice is everywhere. From pop psychology to pop music, from Hallmark to hip-hop, from TED talks to teddy bears, well-being wisdom abounds. But is it real wisdom? If so, what is its basis?

Psychology has a scientific basis, but popular books on the topic tend toward therapeutic tips. Philosophy offers abstract principles ranging from stoicism to hedonism. Poetry and prose give eloquent expression to deeply personal opinions.

This book combines the deeply personal with the massively empirical. Its basis is a gold-standard survey spanning five decades and interviewing

B. J. Jones, *The Pursuit of Happiness in America*, https://doi.org/10.1007/978-3-031-65607-1_1

well over sixty thousand Americans. But before giving the specifications of the book's scientific foundation, consider some proverbial words of wisdom:

> I thank my stars I am happy.
> - Shakespeare
>
> Happiness makes up in height what it lacks in length.
> - Robert Frost
>
> It is neither wealth nor splendor but tranquility and occupation which give you happiness.
> - Thomas Jefferson
>
> There is only one happiness in this life, to love and be loved.
> - George Sand
>
> Most folks are as happy as they make up their minds to be.
> - Abraham Lincoln

Now ponder the content of each aphorism. Shakespeare offers thanks to luck or, in his era, fate. Not very helpful. Robert Frost notes that happiness in all its glory is fleeting. Why is this so? Jefferson seems to suggest that one's occupation is the source of happiness. That might have been his experience, but is it true for non-presidents? Love, certainly, is a reasonable precedent, but how about folks with a tumultuous love life—like George Sand? Finally, it would seem that Abraham Lincoln made up his mind to be, well, depressed and unhappy.

Here is the point. As the Dalai Lama's opening quote states, happiness is important. Important enough, clearly, to be illuminated by real evidence. The General Social Survey is as real as it gets. The project commenced in 1972 with a National Science Foundation grant which has supported its multi-million-dollar budget up through the present day. From the website:

> For five decades, the General Social Survey (GSS) has studied the growing complexity of American society. It is the only *full-probability, personal interview* survey designed to monitor changes in both *social characteristics* and *attitudes* currently being conducted in the United States (italics added).[1]

It is worth unpacking the highlighted phrases to highlight survey quality. "Full probability" is a multistage sampling design that randomly selects smaller and smaller geographical units until it arrives at the household level. One household member is then selected to participate in a "personal interview" asking some 300 questions. These features are known to produce highly representative, premium quality data that can be generalized to the whole U.S. population. They are the reason that GSS results are more accurate than, say, political polls that simply sample area code lists then survey people over the phone. By vivid contrast to the latter, the GSS has had a response rate (the percentage of respondents contacted who agree to be surveyed) in excess of 70%, far surpassing the results for any survey outside of the U.S. census.[2] This level of quality is the reason that the National Opinion Research Center (NORC) administers the survey in such an elaborate manner, and it is also the reason GSS data has been utilized in over 14,000 journal articles and 7500 books. It is certainly good enough—and real enough—evidence for this book.

The "attitudes" referred to in the quote above obviously include those tapping into personal happiness, but "social characteristics" bears some discussion. The phrase is a close relative of "The Sociological Perspective," this book's subtitle which elicits a stark contrast to myriad other volumes on the topic.

Perhaps the best known is the aptly titled *World Happiness Report 2022*, tenth edition. The first edition was commissioned subsequent to United Nations resolution 65/309 to review evidence for the "Defining a New Economic Paradigm" report.[3] As one would expect, the model focuses upon income and other economic variables. The centerpiece is the so-called Cantril Ladder of life evaluation:

> Please imagine a ladder with steps numbered from zero at the bottom to ten at the top. The top of the ladder represents the best possible life for you and the bottom of the ladder represents the worst possible life for you. On which step of the ladder would you say you personally feel you stand at this time?[4]

The Gallup poll asked this (and related) questions in many societies worldwide, then ranked average responses. In this report, Finland was #1 and Afghanistan was #146. Statistical analysis then decomposed the societal factors significantly related to the ladder score. Among five other measures of political economy in the model is "social support," a simple yes/no response to, "If you were in trouble, do you have relatives or friends you can count on to help you whenever you need them, or not?".[5] The analyses below will develop models that are, frankly, much more sociological and zeroed in on the society here ranked #16—that is, America.

Near the top of any list of books about happiness is *The Good Life: Lessons from the World's Longest Study of Happiness.*[6] Authors Robert Waldinger and Marc Schulz are a psychiatrist and a psychologist, respectively. Nevertheless, their central finding borders on the sociological: "Good relationships keep us healthier and happier. Period."[7] The study behind the book is quite remarkable. It commenced in 1938 with a sample of 268 Harvard sophomores and, as a comparison group, 456 12- to 16-year-old boys from inner city Boston. This study is ongoing with some 1300 descendants and spouses in addition to the original participants. Remarkable as it is, no one would take a Harvard/Southie sample to be representative of the entirety of American society. Moreover, the focus is on how satisfied individuals are with their relationships—how warm, strong, and empathetic they *feel* to the respondents. There is some overlap with the present project, but the sociological focus here turns up the magnification on the quantity and quality of the social structures themselves.

Emblematic of the rising tide of interest in well-being research is the very existence of the *Journal of Happiness Studies.* It was founded in 2000 under the auspices of Ruut Veenhoven, a renowned Dutch sociologist. In the "aims and scope" section of its website it states:

> (The journal) covers topics referring to both the hedonic and eudaimonic perspectives characterizing well-being studies. The former includes the investigation of cognitive dimensions such as satisfaction with life and positive affect and emotions. The latter includes the study of constructs and processes related to optimal psychological functioning, such as meaning and purpose in life (emphasis added).

It is certainly useful to conceptualize happiness in the separate dimensions of "hedonic" (positive affect) and "eudaimonic" (meaning and purpose), but again there is the focus on internal—that is, psychological—states. The special sociological contribution of *JHS* is examining international, cross-cultural patterns. The present project spotlights social patterns in the singular society of America.

Measuring Happiness

So, this book will move the vantage point for scrutinizing happiness to the social structures that surround ourselves. That radical change in perspective, though, cannot obviate the need to tap what is called on page one the "deeply personal." Here is the main device for that purpose:

Taken all together, how would you say things are these days – would you say that you are very happy, pretty happy, nor not too happy?

This is a straightforward, simple question. Is it *too* simple? And is there any reason to believe this single question can really measure personal happiness? The answers are no and yes, respectively:

> Despite the simplicity of the happiness measure, there is considerable evidence of its psychometric adequacy in both U.S. and international research. The measure has adequate *validity*. Most people know quite well whether or not they enjoy life … Findings from previous research also show that the measure has considerable *reliability*.[8]

The italicized terms are technical criteria of measurement quality. Validity means that happiness really *is* being tapped, and reliability that repeated measures are consistent. Sociologist Ruut Veenhoven (from above) reports that the GSS happiness item also consistently correlates well with multiple-question indexes of life-satisfaction.[9]

It is time to get "massively empirical," also in the words of page one. Figure 1.1 displays the data distribution of happiness in America over the entire 1972–2018 period. This encompasses thirty-two separate

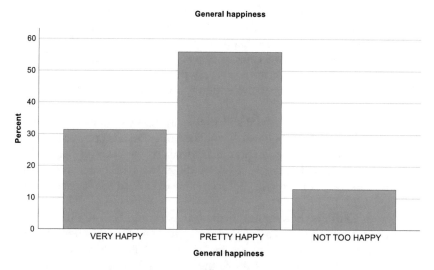

Fig. 1.1 The distribution of happiness in America

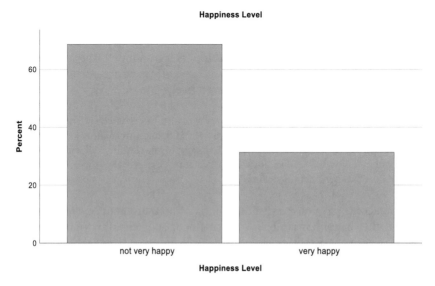

Fig. 1.2   Very happy Americans compared to all others

state-of-the-art samples totaling over 60,000 "deeply personal" responses to the happiness question. The tallest bar in the chart by far is "pretty happy" with 55.9%. 31.3% of Americans have registered "very happy," and only 12.8% have said "not too happy." For most (but not all) of the analyses to come, the latter two categories will be folded together to form a clear counterpoint to Americans who say they are truly happy. Figure 1.2 shows this stark contrast of the roughly one-third highly happy versus everybody else.

The idea, of course, is to distill the sociological sources of that very happy few. Five decades of data offers enormous statistical power to do so, but it also amounts to history. So much social change has swept across this society over recent decades that our findings must be tested over time. Distilled social patterns will be routinely examined on a decade-by-decade basis.

Figure 1.3 offers the simplest form of time testing. GSS administrations have been grouped by decade to smooth out year-to-year variations, and the decades tell a story: happiness in America is down, down, down, and down again. In the 1970s, 34.3% of the population picked the top happiness category, and it declined each decade to 29.2% in the 2010s. If real,

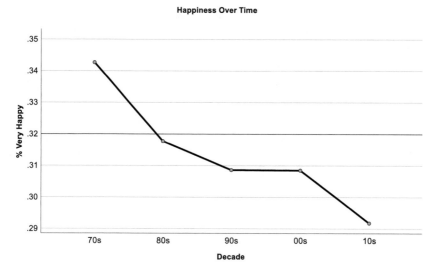

Fig. 1.3 The decline of happiness in America over time

this would be real news. Be reminded that, despite its technical bona fides, the GSS is a sample and not a census. To test the time effect, therefore, inferential statistics are required. That requirement will be fulfilled by ANOVA, the analysis of variance.[10] It is a powerful statistical technique that is a. flexible enough to incorporate different types of variables in the model and b. amenable to visual display for non-specialists; statistical details are available in the footnotes for specialists.[11]

The decade decline in Fig. 1.3 is real or, more formally, statistically significant.[12] It needs to be tested in more complex models which will be previewed now. Figure 1.4 shifts perspective to the following item:

Would you say your own health, in general, is excellent, good, fair, or poor?

So personal health is now on the x-axis—technically, the independent variable—and happiness is in the familiar y-axis, dependent variable position. The appearance of multiple effect lines means that a third variable has been introduced, namely decade. The basic shape of the relationship is obvious in two senses. First, happiness percentage drops at each poorer level of health, and second, no one is surprised that excellent health is

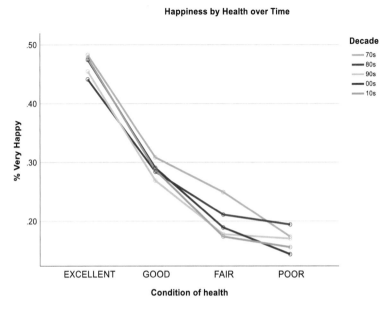

Fig. 1.4 The relationship of health and happiness over time

associated with higher happiness. But something more subtle appears here. Notice that the blue 1970s dots are atop the others, especially at the "fair" and "poor" health levels. The maroon 1980s dots also hover above other decades on the right. ANOVA has a way to tease out such subtle differences. It is known as an interaction effect, and here it means that the effect of health depends on—that is, interacts with—the effect of decade. Quite simply, the downward push of poor health on happiness is stronger lately than it used to be.[13]

THE SOCIOLOGICAL PERSPECTIVE

The choice of physical health to introduce our analytical model was deliberate for two reasons. First, it is a clear, hand-picked illustration of a multivariate effect on happiness. Second, and more to the point, we do not care about this particular effect. It does not pass the non-obvious test— that is, everybody knows that physical suffering can be hard on happiness—and, even more to the point, it does not pass the sociology test. The mission of the present project is to cruise past the sign posts of biology, psychology, and philosophy; to ignore stopping off points in literature and pop culture; to look past celebrity and guru wisdom. Destination: social structure.

IN THEIR OWN WORDS

There is no need to hype the GSS. It is simply the gold standard for quantitative research and, when used in the proper statistical models, the path to accurate generalization about the entire U.S. adult population.[14] But given the unique nature of happiness, statistical breadth is not the only criterion. Probing people's *reasons for* their perceived well-being is a path to adding depth.

In the chapters to follow and immediately below, the results of qualitative interviews will add dimension to the quantitative story. The author commissioned a study by Braun Research Inc., a professional interviewing firm that sampled 50 Americans of diverse genders, ages, races and regions. Their words add personal insight to the expansive reach of the GSS.

The opening question in the qualitative interview is,

> 1. Taken all together, how would you say things are these days -- would you say that you are very happy, pretty happy, or not too happy?
> a.   Why do you say that ... what are the main reasons you would describe yourself as ...?

The first part, of course, simply replicates the GSS item quantified above. Quantification is not the point here, so subpoint 1a probes the *why*. Stacie, a 52-year-old female sales operation manager, says she is pretty happy because, "I have financial stability, a husband that treats me well and good health." Note that her reasons are several, and she even mentions the relevance of health introduced above. Michael, a Native American male teacher, is also pretty happy: "World and national affairs are stressful. I own my own home and I like my job. I have a significant other that I love very much." Again, multiple factors are mentioned, many grounded in the real (social) world. Finally, a 69-year-old white woman cites so many factors that her response needs to be indented:

I own my own house and I feel secure, and I live in California and the weather is nice and I have a garden I enjoy with a nice family and children. I don't have any financial problems, so that is good.

At the other extreme are some folks with burdens so heavy that they give a singular reason for "not too happy." Otis, a 55-year-old white male in Louisiana, is diabetic with fluid in his stomach and heart failure. An 80-year-old retired woman offers only that she has lost her beloved husband and her son as well.

It is notable that the distribution of responses here is *not* a match for the GSS item in two respects. First and most simply, the 16% very happy, 68% pretty happy, and 16% not too happy does not mirror the breakdown in Fig. 1.1 This is because, secondly, a fifty-person qualitative survey is not designed to match the scientific sampling rigor of the General Social Survey. The point, rather, is to enrich abstract numbers with human content. For example, a 44-year-old part-time comedian says he is pretty happy because, "I am still alive and I have everything I can ask for." Along with the darker examples immediately above, these very personal responses provide more emotional dimension than just another check in a box.

The combination of quantitative breadth and qualitative depth has long been acclaimed in sociology. Due to professional specialization and project costs, realization of that potential has been slow. But the time of mixed methods seems to be at hand. Sage Publications now has a *Journal of Mixed Methods Research.* And projects like the present will hopefully offer more proof of concept.

NOTES

1. Smith, Tom W., Davern, Michael, Freese, Jeremy and Morgan, Stephen L., General Social Surveys 1972–2018 [machine readable data file]/Principal Investigator, Smith, Tom W.; Co-Principal Investigator, Michael Davern, Jeremy Freese and Stephen L. Morgan; sponsored by National Science Foundation -- NORC ed. -- Chicago: NORC, 2019. 1 data file (64, 814 logical records + 1 codebook (3758 pp.). -- (National Data Program for the Social Sciences, no. 25).
2. John Robinson. General Social Survey (GSS): USA. In: Michalos, A.C. (ed) *Encyclopedia of Quality of Life and Well-Being Research.* (Springer: Dordrecht, 2014).
3. Helliwell, J.F., Layard, R., Sachs, J.D., De Neve, J.E., Aknin, L.B., & Wang, S. (Eds.). *World Happiness Report* 2022 (New York: Sustainable Development Solutions Network, 2022), 7.

4. Cantril, H., *The Pattern of Human Concerns* (New Brunswick, N.J.: Rutgers University Press, 1965).
5. Helliwell et al., op. cit., 21.
6. Robert Waldinger and Marc Schulz, *The Good Life: Lessons from the World's Longest Study of Happiness* (New York: Simon & Schuster, 2023).
7. Ibid., 3.
8. Yang Yang, "Long and Happy Living: Trends and Patterns of Happy Life Expectancy in the U.S., 19700-2000," *Social Science Research* (2008, Vol. 37), p. 1239.
9. Ruut Veenhoven, "Developments in Satisfaction Research," *Social Indicators Research* (January 1996, Vol. 37), 1–46.
10. Stehlik-Barry and Anthony J. Babinec, *Data Analysis with IBM SPSS Statistics: Implementing Data Modeling, Descriptive Statistics and ANOVA* (Birmingham, UK: Packt Publishing, 2017).
11. Specialists will be interested to know that happiness has a 0 vs. 1 code to satisfy the intervality assumption of ANOVA.
12. For the main effect of decade, $F = 17.917$, $p < 0.001$.
13. For the main effect of health, $F = 759.912$, $p < 0.001$; for the interaction effect, $F = 2.482$, $p = 0.003$.
14. The GSS samples adults 18 and older, and the estimated sampling error is between 2 and 3 percent.

References

Cantril, H., *The Pattern of Human Concerns* (New Brunswick, N.J.: Rutgers University Press, 1965).

Helliwell, J.F., R. Layard, J.D. Sachs, J.E De Neve, L.B. Aknin, and S. Wang (Eds.). *World Happiness Report 2022* (New York: Sustainable Development Solutions Network, 2022).

Robinson, John. General Social Survey (GSS): USA. In: A.C. Michalos (ed.) *Encyclopedia of Quality of Life and Well-Being Research.* (Springer: Dordrecht, 2014).

Stehlik-Barry, Kenneth and Anthony J. Babinec, *Data Analysis with IBM SPSS Statistics: Implementing Data Modeling, Descriptive Statistics and ANOVA* (Birmingham, UK: Packt Publishing, 2017).

Veenhoven, Ruut, "Developments in Satisfaction Research," *Social Indicators Research* (January 1996, Vol. 37), 1-46.

Waldinger, Robert, and Marc Schulz, *The Good Life: Lessons from the World's Longest Study of Happiness* (New York: Simon & Schuster, 2023).

Yang, Yang, "Long and Happy Living: Trends and Patterns of Happy Life Expectancy in the U.S., 19700–2000," *Social Science Research* (2008, Vol. 37).

CHAPTER 2

Pillars of Happiness: Attitudes

Abstract The present chapter takes a social psychological approach by spotlighting attitudes related to happiness. Americans very satisfied with their jobs are much more likely to be very happy. Americans very happy with their marriages are very much more likely to be very happy. Both of these relationships link social structures (i.e., jobs and marriages) to personal happiness, and both relationships have endured across five decades.

Keywords Job satisfaction • Marital happiness

Given the clarion call of Chap. 1 for attention to social structures, the above title warrants some explanation. "Attitudes" would seem to be the province of psychology, but consider a recent Wikipedia entry:

> Social psychology is the scientific study of how thoughts, feelings, and behaviors are influenced by the real or imagined presence of other people or by social norms ... (it studies) the social conditions under which thoughts, feelings, and behaviors occur, and how these variables influence social interactions.

So, a particular subset of attitudes are to be scrutinized here—those with social connections.

B. J. Jones, *The Pursuit of Happiness in America*, https://doi.org/10.1007/978-3-031-65607-1_2

The use of "pillars" likewise bears comment. Take a moment to think about your current level of happiness. As you turn it over in your mind, inevitably a kind of check list pops up. Is the career on track? How is my family life? The answers to such questions would seem to support overall happiness. "Would seem" is a conditional statement which now will be subject to empirical analysis.

JOB SATISFACTION

Americans love their jobs. This is a truism that turns out to be true. Figure 2.1 offers evidence in response to the following GSS item:

> On the whole, how satisfied are you with the work you do—would you say you are very satisfied, moderately satisfied, a little dissatisfied, or very dissatisfied?

The figure shows that a full 48% give the "very satisfied response," very nearly matching all other responses combined. It has been recoded into this simplified form to parallel the main happiness question and, like the latter, is a single item tapping a complex part of life. After all, a professor might love teaching but detest the grading that it requires. But the studies

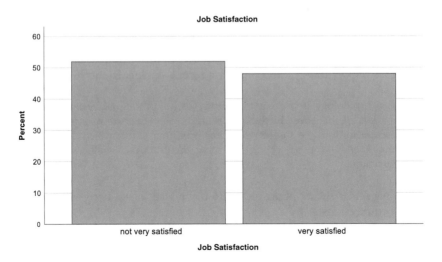

Fig. 2.1 Job satisfaction in America

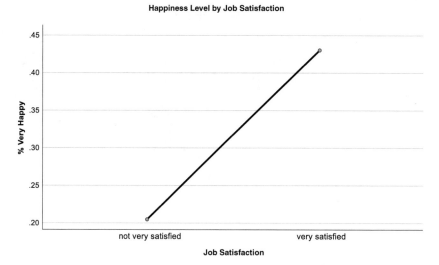

Fig. 2.2 Americans very satisfied with their jobs are much more likely to be very happy

are clear: overall job satisfaction questions like this relate consistently well to multidimensional work measures.[1] People do have a general attitude about their jobs.

But does happy at work mean happy in general? Figure 2.2 gives an affirmative answer. Americans who are very satisfied with their work have a 43% likelihood of being very happy compared to 20.5% for those with lesser job satisfaction. This is such a steep difference that formal statistical testing is superfluous.[2] One can *more than double* their chance of high happiness with high job satisfaction. It is easy to visualize the right-hand top point being supported by, well, a pillar.

Both the ups and downs of the U.S. economy and common sense call for scrutiny of this relationship by decade. Figure 2.3 does so with striking results. One is first struck by the steep elevation of happiness above "very satisfied" in every decade. So a strong main effect of job satisfaction has been a constant, but ANOVA's routine tests discern two less apparent relations. Note first that the blue 1970s dots are atop all other decades. This is the substance of a downward shift in overall happiness (a finding previewed in Chap. 1), but there is a more nuanced change as well. The dots at right drop a bit in each decade such that the 2010s (GSS

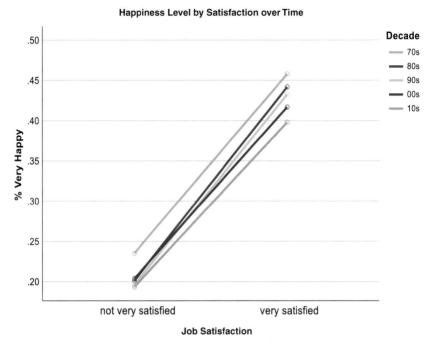

Fig. 2.3 The relationship of job satisfaction and happiness has endured over time

administrations 2010 through 2018) are at the bottom. This significant interaction effect translates to a lesser—but still formidable—impact of job satisfaction on happiness over time.[3]

MARITAL HAPPINESS

To echo the start of the previous section: Americans love their spouses, too. Here is how the GSS poses the question:

> Taking all things together, how would you describe your marriage? Would you say that your marriage is very happy, pretty happy, or not too happy?[4]

Figure 2.4 displays very happy marriages (63.3%) towering over the other responses combined (36.7%). The careful reader will have noted the similarity of wording to the general happiness question, but more is at play in

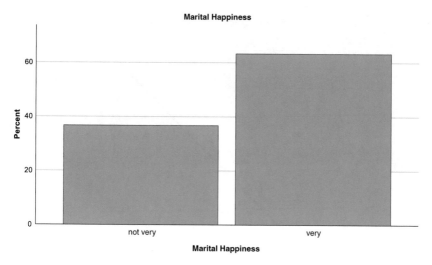

Fig. 2.4 Marital happiness in America

Fig. 2.5 than verbal mimicry. A full 57.9% of Americans with very happy marriages are also very happy; by comparison, the very happy share for Americans with less happy marriages is a paltry 11.1%. This titanic difference has endured over time. In Fig. 2.6, observe the nearly perfect parallelism of the lines for each decade. The lines, of course, simply connect the dot percentages which here cluster together. ANOVA confirms both the size and the persistence of the marital happiness effect.[5]

It is worth pausing to ponder this recent spate of findings. Job and marriage are stalwart pillars of personal happiness, full stop. These are not free-floating attitudes. Each is specifically tied to a concrete social structure. And they are both part of everyday American lives. To return for a moment to aphorisms, Sigmund Freud's famous quote is "Love and work are the cornerstone of our humanness." We can now substitute pillars for cornerstones, happiness for humanness, and sociological evidence for psychological observation.

The sociological perspective also offers a deeper dive. Figure 2.7 breaks down the effects of job and marital satisfaction to observe their independent operation. One might speculate that happy folks are just happy folks and their joint experience in these separate social domains would make no

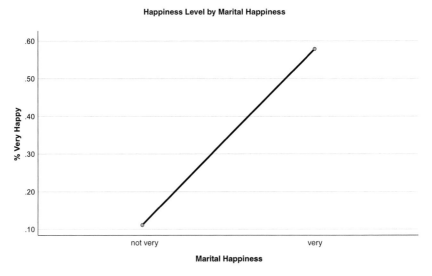

Fig. 2.5 Americans very happy with their marriages are much more likely to be very happy

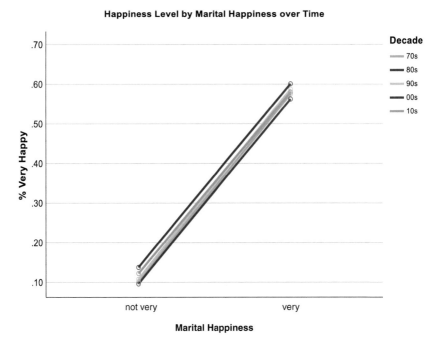

Fig. 2.6 The relationship of marital happiness and happiness has endured over time

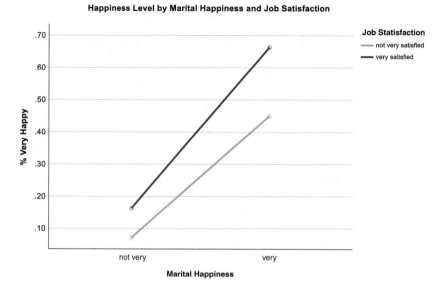

Fig. 2.7 Job satisfaction and marital happiness have independent effects on happiness

difference. Data trump speculation. Observe how steeply the dot averages rise to the right. Also observe the significant separation between the red and blue dots. Translation: marital happiness elevates personal happiness regardless of job satisfaction level and—given the separation—job satisfaction matters, too, for both levels of marital satisfaction. One may also discern that the slope of the red, high job satisfaction, line is noticeably greater. To wit: marital happiness is associated with an even greater happiness surge for Americans who love their jobs.[6]

The formidable time span and sample size covered by these findings call for a breakdown by decade. Doing so (analysis not shown) just reinforces our above conclusions. Each social psychological attitude has a significant singular effect on overall happiness, and the dual marital happiness—job satisfaction effect comes through as well. Furthermore, a separate statistical test of whether the scale of these effects changed substantively over time was negative.[7] Over the recent social history of U.S. society, good marriages and good jobs have been pillars of the good life.

In Their Own Words

The whole idea of qualitative research is to use open-ended questions which allow people to answer, well, in their own words. Items like the following are truly unbounded:

> 2. What would you say are the major factors in your life that make you happy? Could you give me some examples?

The very openness of the question allows people to volunteer answers without prompting. Several folks went right to marriage and work together. Retirement-age male civil prosecutor Thomas responds, "I am married to a wonderful woman. I have a good job." A thirty-something Philadelphia hair stylist is more expansive:

> I work with really good people and my job is not extremely hard and I am not too stressed out at work. I have a good family that helps out with the baby and I have a happy marriage …

Many of the fifty respondents mention *either* work *or* a spouse/partner as a major happiness source. By actual count it is sixteen of each, further justifying the two focal points of this chapter.

By no means are these the only two "major factors." Twenty percent of the survey sample mention pets. The civil prosecutor quoted above also says, "I have two dogs and three cats I enjoy." To the above the hair stylist adds, "and I have a dog who is ten years old and doing good." The stock phrase "family and friends" is the next most common; an unmarried operational manager from West Virginia actually previews Chap. 4 by offering, "My relationships with people gives me the most satisfaction." A handful of respondents cite religion, one 911 operator from Georgia giving this reason: "Being able to go to church and feel the spirit and know there is a loving god out there."

The follow-up question is the natural real-world counterpart to #2:

> 3. Now let me ask about the other side of things. What would you say are the major factors in your life that contribute to making you less happy? Could you give me some examples?

Michael, a high school teacher from South Carolina has an omnibus answer:

I do experience loss when loved ones and family members die … Stuff in the world like politics. I am 34 and there is a part of me that thought I would be married and have kids … Money; I have everything I need, but personally I have too much credit card debt and there is too much inflation … I struggle with losing weight. I am never happy with my body and my fitness level.

Despite this list, Michael claims to be "pretty happy," and his list identifies themes in the pattern of responses.

One real surprise is the number of people mirroring Michael's "stuff in the world like politics" response. No fewer than sixteen respondents cited political issues. A retired white woman from Greece, New York, says, "The political situation right now and the lying and cheating that is going on. We are turning into a fascist country." RJS, a 63-year-old male engineer from Wisconsin offers, "On a bigger scale beyond family, the political environment of the country has raised concern." Remember, these folks are not just saying that political issues are on their mind, but that they are "major factors" bearing on their unhappiness.

About half a dozen responses center on economic issues. The major factor for a maintenance man from Norwood, Massachusetts is, "All around prices of everything—the economy." An unemployed 44-year-old bi-racial female in Baltimore replies with a personal epigram: "They say that money doesn't buy happiness. They are wrong. Not having money has made me decidedly less happy."

But the most prominent set of negative happiness concerns involves family members. Along with Michael, a number deeply feel the loss of relatives. An 80-year-old widow from Hughson, Nevada simply says, "I don't have my husband here. He was the love of my life." Heartbreak is real, and it can extend to ongoing health issues. One 88-year-old black man from Chicago reports, "My wife is still with me after 56 years … she has dementia." A 48-year-old female legal assistant in Greensboro, North Carolina cites "Overwhelming stress due to poor health of other family members." Some happiness-draining factors involve relationships with family members. The Wisconsin engineer quoted above here volunteers that "Raising children can be challenging." An elderly black woman from Massachusetts is concerned that, "Sometimes you expect more out of your husband than they give."

No simple summary can do justice to these multiple factors adding to and subtracting from happiness. It is worthwhile to note, though, that the inner self is not the major source. Quite a few folks do suffer from physical and psychological conditions, but most factors freely offered reside, to use a phrase oft-repeated here, in the real social world.

NOTES

1. Felix Requena, "Social Capital, Satisfaction and Quality of Life in the Workplace," *Social Indicators Research* (July 2002, Vol. 61), 331–360. Yoav Gonzarch, "Intelligence, Education and Facets of Job Satisfaction," *Work and Organizations* (2003, Vol. 30), 97–112. Lori J. Ducharme and Jack K. Martin, "Unrewarding Work, Coworker Support and Job Satisfaction: A Test of the Buffering Hypothesis," *Work and Occupations* (2000, Vol. 27), 223–243.

2. Nevertheless, specialists may seek statistical confirmation. $F = 2890.206$, $p < 0.001$.

3. For the main effect of job satisfaction, $F = 2787.222$, $p < 0.001$; for the main effect of decade, $F = 14.322$, $p < 0.001$; for the interaction effect, $F = 2.749$, $p = 0.027$.

4. This single item has proven to be a serviceable measure of overall marital quality. Claire M. Kamp Dush, Miles G. Taylor and Rhiannon A. Koreger, "Marital Happiness and Psychological Well-Being across the Life Course," *Family Relations* (2008, Vol. 57), 211–226.

5. For the main effect of marital happiness, $F = 7903.625$, $p < 0.001$; for the interaction effect, $F = 0.518$, $p = $ n.s.

6. For the main effect of marital happiness, $F = 5962.775$, $p < 0.001$; for the main effect of job satisfaction, $F = 715.605$, $p < 0.001$; for the interaction effect, $F = 115.066$, $p < 0.001$.

7. The main effect of marital happiness and job satisfaction as well as their interaction effect remained statistically significant. For the interaction effect of marital happiness-job satisfaction-decade, $F = 0.637$, $p = $ n.s.

REFERENCES

Ducharme, Lori J., and Jack K. Martin, "Unrewarding Work, Coworker Support and Job Satisfaction: A Test of the Buffering Hypothesis," *Work and Occupations* (2000, Vol. 27).

Dush, Claire M. Kamp, Miles G. Taylor, and Rhiannon A. Koreger, "Marital Happiness and Psychological Well-Being across the Life Course," *Family Relations* (2008, Vol. 57).

Gonzarch, Yoav, "Intelligence, Education and Facets of Job Satisfaction," *Work and Organizations* (2003, Vol. 30).

Requena, Felix "Social Capital, Satisfaction and Quality of Life in the Workplace," *Social Indicators Research* (July 2002, Vol. 61).

CHAPTER 3

Sources of Happiness: Social Structures

Abstract Here the focus is directly on social structures and happiness. By being married Americans double their chances of being very happy. Subjective social class is positively associated with happiness independently of family income. Network socializing is positively associated with happiness, especially for older Americans.

Keywords Marriage • Subjective social class • Network socializing

It is worth wondering why we began with evidence about attitudes concerning social structures rather than the social structures themselves. The answer is simple: credibility. To establish the relevance of a factor to personal functioning, it is reasonable to test its extremes. Psychologists sold the concept of stress by developing an entire literature on traumatic life events. This highest level of distress helped establish the importance of stress generally. Likewise, it is now clear that social structures are generally germane to personal happiness.

© The Author(s), under exclusive license to Springer Nature Switzerland AG 2024
B. J. Jones, *The Pursuit of Happiness in America*,
https://doi.org/10.1007/978-3-031-65607-1_3

MARRIAGE

Taking the lead to move beyond the prima facie case for social structure will be marital status. The GSS item offers five responses: married, widowed, divorced, separated, and never married. For maximum comparative clarity, the last four were collapsed creating a married/unmarried dichotomy.

Figure 3.1 could not be more clear. Americans married at survey time show a much greater likelihood of high happiness than the unmarried. Across the five decades, marriage roughly doubles the chance of being very happy, 40.4% to 21.1%. This is remarkable for (at least) three reasons. Reason one shadows the argument above. Level of marital happiness is an unmeasured variable here so Fig. 3.1 displays the potent effect of the *mere fact* of being married.[1] Second, this effect exists for males and females, for blacks and whites, for young and old; indeed, for every variable the author has conceived of and tested. The final reason is most remarkable given the other two: marriage in America is in precipitous decline. That is the minimal description of the trend line in Fig. 3.2. To specify it a bit, at the first GSS in 1972, 71.9% of Americans were married; by the final administration here in 2018, the number had dived to 42.5%. Precipitous indeed.

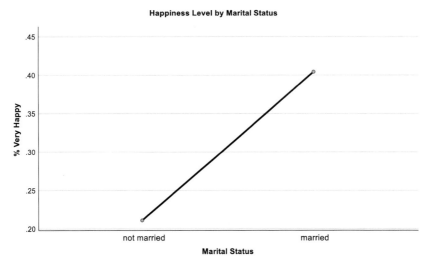

Fig. 3.1 Married Americans are much more likely to be very happy than unmarried Americans

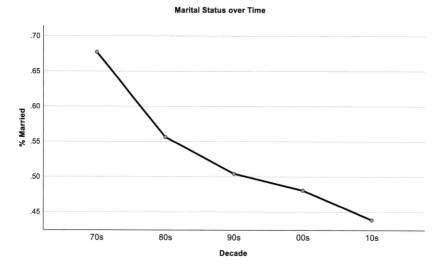

Fig. 3.2 The decline of marriage in America

So there has been a society-wide abandonment of a social structure despite its apparent felicitous effects. This paradox calls to mind the society-wide drop in happiness documented in Fig. 1.3. At that time, "more complex models" were promised to unravel its sources. Figure 3.3 now fulfills some of that promise. The insertion of marriage into the long-term trend analysis in effect erases the long-term trend. Aside from minor decade-to-decade oscillations, the percent-very-happy averages barely budge within marital statuses. For unmarried Americans, 20.9% were very happy in the 1970s compared to 20.3% in the most recent decade; for married Americans, the respective percentages are 40.6% and 40.5%. Additional complexities are to come, but one simple conclusion fits these facts: when marital status is statistically controlled, the decade decline in American happiness disappears.[2]

There is one complexity that needs be confronted now. All statistical tests presented so far are estimates of *association*, that is, of some relationship between variables. It borders on methodological cliché to not mistake such data for evidence of *causation*. It is worth raising the cliché in this case because of a perfectly plausible question: who gets married? Reasonable response: happy people. Upbeat folks might be more attractive to others, and more disposed to seek out others, as well. This is not a straw man to

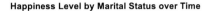

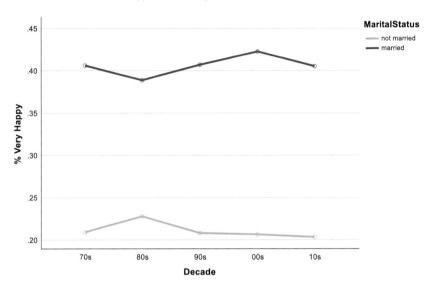

Fig. 3.3   Within marital statuses there has been no decline in happiness in America

be cast aside with some dismissive argument. In fact, Chap. 7 will use a special GSS panel to present evidence about which way the causal arrow runs—from marriage to happiness or, to the above point, happiness to marriage.

Social Class

Social structure is a big idea. It encompasses familiar, personally constructed connections—such as marriage—and reaches right up to the very idea of society itself.

At an intermediary level in this expansive range is social class. The concept has roots in sociology stretching back to (at least) Karl Marx and Max Weber, and it has everyday resonance in American life. One marker of its presence in modern sociology is a much-cited source, *Social Stratification: Class, Race and Gender in Sociological Perspective*; it is composed of 32 edited articles and some 1100 pages.[3] Despite this (literal) weight of scholarship, another major source to be considered here is entitled *Social Class: How Does it Work?* One might suppose that the raw tonnage of scholarship would have settled such a basic question, but no. According to the editors of the latter volume, "considerable murkiness swirls around the empirical study of social class" and so "we should embrace a folk concept of class."[4] From literary folklore comes the following dialogue:

> F. Scott Fitzgerald: "The rich are different than you and me."
> Ernest Hemingway: "Yes - they have more money."

Apocryphal or not, this famous exchange lays bare a key question about social class: is it about more than money?

Despite all the hand-wringing by professional sociologists, Americans themselves seem to have no trouble at all identifying their social class. The GSS poses this simple question:

> *If you were asked to use one of these four names for your social class, which would you say you belong in? Upper class, middle class, working class, or lower class?*

According to Michael Hout of Berkeley, 99% of respondents readily identify with one of these four categories.[5] It is a subjective question, contrasting with the more technical objective categories superimposed by sociologists.[6]

Figure 3.4 dives right into the Fitzgerald-Hemingway, subjective-objective class question. On the x-axis are the categories of the subjective social class item, left to right: lower class, working class, middle class, and upper class. Percent very happy is in its familiar y-axis position, but something objective has been added: family income, adjusted for inflation due to the time span of the data.[7] Note first that average happiness rises with income at each class level. Money does matter regardless of class position. But the more pertinent point is how decisive class is even with income statistically controlled. The very happy dot averages rise at each income level approximately 20% from lower to upper class. Also observe how suspiciously linear the effects are.[8] Fitzgerald would seem to be right, but for every class rung, not just the rich.

These findings make a strong case for our common sense measure of social class, but there is a further argument for social structure. In Fig. 3.5, job satisfaction is on the dependent variable axis. Despite the obvious importance of salary and wages, the class ladder elevates job satisfaction at each rung and at each income level.[9] This figure displays another highly linear class effect, net of money.

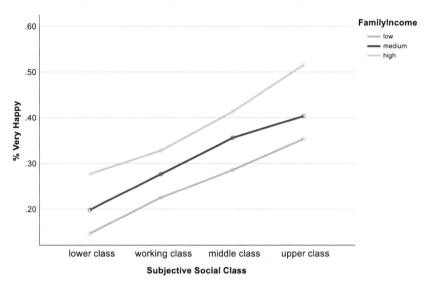

Fig. 3.4 Subjective social class and family income have independent effects on happiness

Since the box for Chap. 2 has already been opened, we now turn our attention to marriage. The marital happiness averages by class in Fig. 3.6 are, again, strongly positive and suspiciously linear.[10] But we know that there have been dynamic changes in marriage itself—the pure social structure—over recent social history.

Figure 3.7 presents a class-based model of those dynamics. There are confirmations and revelations. The dots representing percent married plummet in every decade for all but the rich, confirming widespread marital decline. But the rate of decline is class-specific. The net change is minus 23% for the lower class, minus 28% for the working class, minus 17.9% for the middle class, and minus 3.1% for the upper class. This alters the very shape of the class-marriage relationship. In the 1970s, the dots traced out a heap in the working class-middle class center with lower percentages at the top and bottom. In the 2010s, the greater attenuation of marriage in the lower and (especially) working classes gradually formed the now-familiar, very-nearly linear relationship.

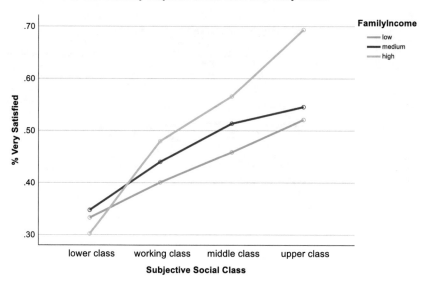

Fig. 3.5 Subjective social class and family income have independent effects on job satisfaction

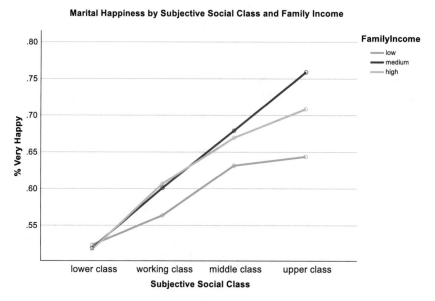

Fig. 3.6 Subjective social class and family income have independent effects on marital happiness

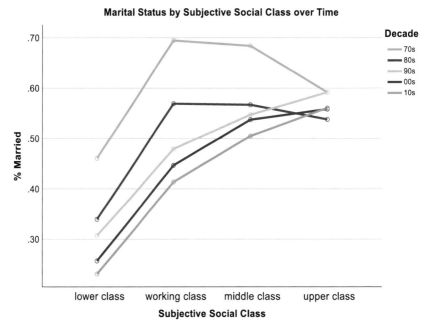

Fig. 3.7   The decline of marriage in America has been class-specific

The revelation, therefore, is twofold. First, class has demonstrated a quasi-linear association with happiness itself and both happiness-related attitudes. Second, over time, subjective class has developed a similar relationship with marriage, clearly linking two important social structures.

Network Socializing

The pursuit of happiness is not conceived as a solitary path. Virtually everyone's vision of that journey involves the company of one's fellows, the modern term for which is social networks. The latter phrase is so well-known it has become a gerund ("networking"), and it is conceived in various ways. The present conception will take advantage of the society-spanning width and historical depth of the GSS using the following set of items:

How often do you spend a social evening with …
… friends who live outside your neighborhood?

… relatives?
… someone who lives in your neighborhood?

0. never
1. about once a year
2. several times a year
3. about once a month
4. several times a month
5. once or twice a week
6. almost every day

So these are measures of frequency of interaction with several notable features. First, the "spend a social evening" wording means that this is a substantive face-to-face interaction, not just a cell phone call or an impromptu talk with a neighbor in the driveway. Second, each item taps a well-known, everyday network category—friend, relative, or neighbor. Third, for present purposes the 0–6 responses are to be totaled across the three categories to produce a 0–18 scale of overall network interaction frequency.[11]

Figure 3.8 simplifies the scale into low, medium, and high levels of network socializing. The association with percent very happy is statistically

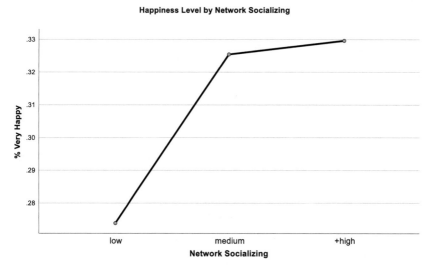

Happiness Level by Network Socializing

Fig. 3.8 Network socializing is positively associated with happiness

significant,[12] and most of the effect occurs in the space between low and medium. The latter category would equate to seeing all three types of network members monthly or two of them weekly, as examples. Moving to the highest level of interaction makes little difference, so it would appear that there is a threshold effect.

For the moment the question of causal direction is tabled, but there is a pressing complication to be considered: age. It is well-established that as Americans get older they both go out less and get happier. Untangling this intersection of effects is the task of Fig. 3.9. It offers an answer in the form of an interaction effect (statistical) about social interaction (actual). The low to medium dog-leg relation is apparent for all three age groups, but the range of happiness spanned by older Americans is clearly greater.[13] Later in the life cycle, people spend fewer social evenings (observe the vertical distance between the dots), but with greater impact on their levels of happiness.

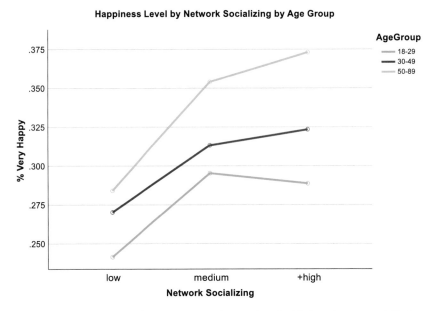

Fig. 3.9 Network socializing is positively associated with happiness especially for older Americans

IN THEIR OWN WORDS

How has your marriage contributed to your happiness? Can you give me some examples?

This is a pointed question. The phrasing is rooted in the causal complexity raised above. Whichever way the causal arrow runs from marriage to happiness, here real people are asked to specify the real benefits they get from their spouses.

Previously, the responses reviewed for this section have been grouped to find common patterns. This does not seem possible here. Folks have offered statements that are singular, personalized, and multiple.

First up is Stacie from Hurst, Texas:

> I have someone who believes in me and has faith in me and is always there when needed. When I am sick, there is someone to take care of me and when I am down, he makes me smile and I have someone there to fight battles for me.

Her statement is not elegant, but it is eloquent in its expression of concrete help with life's difficulties. Perhaps the ultimate perspective is offered by a 99-year-old woman in Sacramento, California:

> The fact that we have built our life around our values. Serious illness has separated us. The fact that we are married and happy together, we are not happy separated. The fact that we get along and we have many things in common like religion, family and togetherness.

In this case, the intrusion of illness has put the long-standing happiness sources of the marriage in bold relief.

Classification of these responses seems unwise both because they are multifaceted and because they are unique. Consider the statement of a white male civil prosecutor:

> My wife is a wonderful, brilliant person and that makes things interesting. I have been married for 34 years. We go places and have family events we go to and have friends. My wife and I are in the same profession and we have lots to talk about … We go on great vacations and have fun going to movies and go out to dinner and have fun with our exchange students.

On the other hand, some statements are simple but no less heartfelt. A 29-year-old Asian statistical programmer mainly appreciates that her husband, "stuck by me, even in emotional moments" and "he came to a lot of therapy sessions." And the 44-year-old male comedian says his wife contributes to his happiness simply because, "She keeps me in line. It is great."

This chapter introduced the concept of class as a social structure. But to use somewhat less academic terminology, the qualitative question was worded as follows:

> How has your economic position contributed to your happiness? Can you give me some examples?

As expected, people think less in terms of general concepts than of everyday coping. According to a male salesman, "I would say greatly, it really does help. Money doesn't buy happiness, but it does sustain you. It causes less stress and worries and opens up opportunities to explore new life experiences." Reducing "stress and worries" is a theme in the responses. A middle-aged Native American teacher says, "I am more relaxed. I am not rich but I am comfortable … I can go out to eat and go to the theater and not have to worry about making my bills."

Several respondents spoke in terms of properly managing the rewards of their economic position. Steve, a law enforcement officer from Joshua Tree, California, puts it this way: "I have invested well and didn't spend it (money) on frivolous stuff and am doing well when I am almost 50." An architectural designer from Portland, Oregon, says,

> There is satisfaction in saving money effectively. I wouldn't say I have a high salary, just saving every penny I have when others would not be able to manage … it all adds up to saving money for the future which … makes me happier.

A few of the respondents are coping with the exigencies of poverty, clearly at the bottom of the class structure. A manufacturing supervisor from Cleveland says economic position "has a heavy effect on whether I am happy … When I lost my job and it took six months to find a new one I could see the impact it had on me." As a counterpoint, Aimee, who works at a bookstore in Crystal River, Florida, offers that, "My economic position has contributed to my happiness because my job is a dream job to me."

NOTES

1. For the main effect of marital status, $F = 27.2.200$, $p < 0.001$.
2. For the main effect of decade with marital status controlled, $F = 0.754$, $p = $ n.s.; for the main effect of marital status with decade controlled, $F = 2631.441$, $p < 0.001$. Using the same dataset but a different scaling of the happiness item, Sam Peltzman reached a similar conclusion. See *The Socio Political Demography of Happiness*, George J. Stigler Center for the Study of the Economy & State, Working Paper No. 331(July 12, 2023), 7–8.
3. David B. Grusky, editor, *Social Stratification: Class, Race and Gender in Sociological Perspective* (Westview Press, 2014).
4. Annette Lareau and Dalton Conley, editors, *Social Class: How Does It Work?* (Russell Sage Foundation, 2008). Pps. 4–5 and 367.
5. Michael Hout, "How Class Works: Objective and Subjective Aspects of Class, since the 1970s," *Social Class: How Does it Work?*, ibid., *29*.
6. Nevertheless, the evidence is strong that this measure correlates very well with objective measures. Michael Hout, "How Class Works," ibid., 32.
7. Variable CONINC has been included in the GSS since 1988. The adjusted categories are lower = \$363–\$23,595, medium = \$23,847–\$49, 883 and high = \$50,295–\$180,386.
8. For the main effect of CONINC, $F = 50.791$, $p < 0.001$; for the main effect of class, $F = 135.139$, $p < 0.001$.
9. For the main effect of class, $F = 90.231$, $p < 0.001$.
10. For the main effect of class, $F = 82.433$, $p < 0.001$.
11. Formally, these are not interval measures but they are judged to be numeric enough to satisfy the intervality assumption. The total scale values were recoded to 3–10 low, 11–13 medium and 14–21 = high.
12. For the main effect of network socializing $F = 56.337$, $p < 0.001$.
13. For the main effect of network socializing, $F = 52.358$, $p < 0.001$; for the interaction effect of age and network socializing, $F = 2.953$, $p = 0.019$.

REFERENCES

Grusky, David B., editor, *Social Stratification: Class, Race and Gender in Sociological Perspective* (Westview Press, 2014).

Hout, Michael, "How Class Works: Objective and Subjective Aspects of Class, since the 1970s," *Social Class: How Does it Work?*.

Lareau, Annette, and Dalton Conley, editors, *Social Class: How Does It Work?* (New York, NY: Russell Sage Foundation, 2008).

CHAPTER 4

"With a Little Help from My …"

Abstract In this chapter the structural elements of network socializing are deconstructed. To be properly understood, these elements must be analyzed within marital statuses. Friend socializing, relative socializing, and neighbor socializing all are positively associated with happiness among married and unmarried Americans. To be properly understood, trends in these network elements must be analyzed within age groups. Friend socializing in America has been on the rise. Relative socializing dipped after the 1970s, but has surged since. Neighbor socializing has dropped significantly across all age groups.

Keywords Friend socializing • Relative socializing • Neighbor socializing

Everyone knows how to complete this line from the Beatles' tune, but it is left dangling for a reason. In addition to friends, relatives and neighbors might help Americans achieve happiness. Here it is an empirical rather than a lyrical question.

B. J. Jones, *The Pursuit of Happiness in America*,
https://doi.org/10.1007/978-3-031-65607-1_4

NETWORK SOCIALIZING AND HAPPINESS

Nevertheless, Fig. 4.1 starts with friend socializing in the whole array of levels from never to daily. The dot averages trace out a surprise. Intermediate friending levels top out those very happy with considerably less happiness at low and high levels. This reverse U-shape tempts premature interpretation. For instance, one might suppose that more friend time helps happiness up to a point, and that beyond several times a month unhappy folks are communing more with friends to get "a little help." Before re-raising the causality complication, turn immediately to Fig. 4.2 which clears up the matter.

The "reverse U-shape" is gone. Instead, there is a discernible upward swing of high happiness by friend socializing for both marital statuses. For married folks, daily interactors are about 10% happier than nevers; for the unmarried, it is about 5%.[1] Moreover, both the direct friending effect and the greater married-friending effect have remained unchanged over time.[2]

This bit of multivariate magic has a ready, everyday explanation. It is a commonplace that married people go out less[3]; it is an empirical fact that married people tend to be happier (see above). Therefore, the downturn

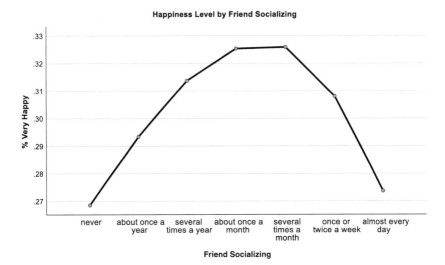

Fig. 4.1 The curvilinear relationship of friend socializing and happiness

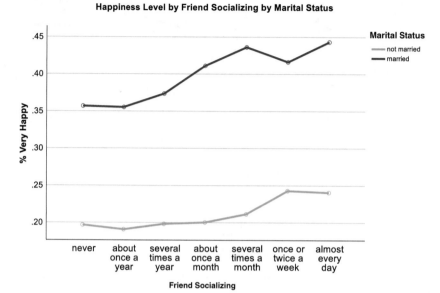

Fig. 4.2 Within marital statuses friend socializing is positively associated with happiness

in Fig. 4.1 is the confluence of less happy but more friend-active unmarrieds. When the marital statuses are statistically separated, both show a positive friend socializing-high happiness connection.

Further confirmation is forthcoming in Figs. 4.3 and 4.4. High levels of evenings spent with relatives and neighbors both display a distinct downturn at high happiness levels (not shown), and both resolve into the familiar pattern when marital status is shown. Marrieds and unmarrieds are at their happiest when relative socializing is high, and even more so for married Americans.[4] Despite a bit of a downturn at the very highest level of socializing for marrieds, the pattern is also there for neighboring.[5]

So to no one's real surprise, socializing and happiness do go together. It is somewhat surprising that socializing magnifies the pro-happiness effect of marriage. But here a change of perspective is in order. Do you think of your network members as tools of your personal happiness? Of course not.

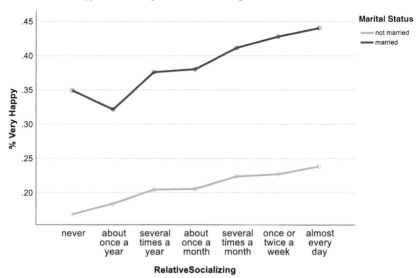

Fig. 4.3 Within marital statuses relative socializing is positively associated with happiness

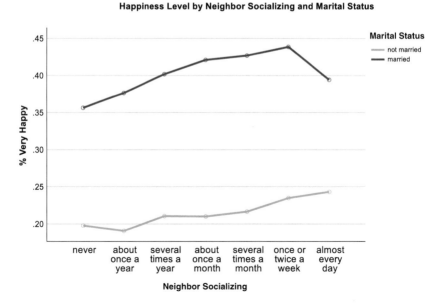

Fig. 4.4 Within martial statuses neighbor socializing is positively associated with happiness

Network Socializing over Time

The point of that provocative ending was to highlight the intrinsic value of personal relationships. Whatever the happiness effects, network socializing can be a joy for its own sake.

So Fig. 4.5 introduces a change of empirical perspective. Friend socializing is now on the y-axis to be tracked over the decades. If Americans are spending less time with their friends over time, something precious has been lost. They have, in fact, been spending more such time, although the increase has trailed off lately.[6] But the end of Chap. 3 proved that age must be taken into account, especially in an era which proclaims the "Graying of America." Figure 4.6 pays off that account. Friending is clearly up in all three age groups, especially among younger and older adults. For the latter, the interaction averages in the 1970s and 1980s have moved upward from "about once a month" toward "several times a month".[7] Friendship is one of the good things in life, and there is indeed more of it in contemporary America.

Socializing with relatives has traced out a different path. For all three age groups in Fig. 4.7 the averages declined from the 1970s into the

Friend Socializing over Time
4.100
4.075
4.050
4.025
4.000
3.975
Friend Socializing
70s
80s
90s
00s
10s
Decade

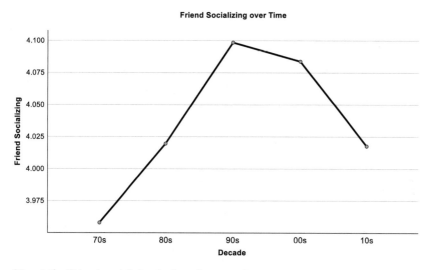

Fig. 4.5 Friend socializing in America over time

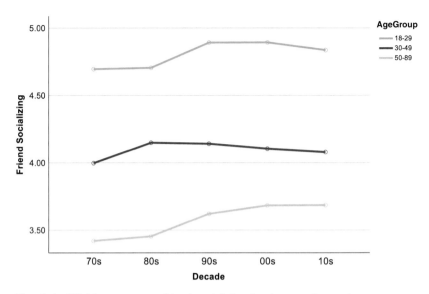

Fig. 4.6 Within age groups friend socializing has increased over time

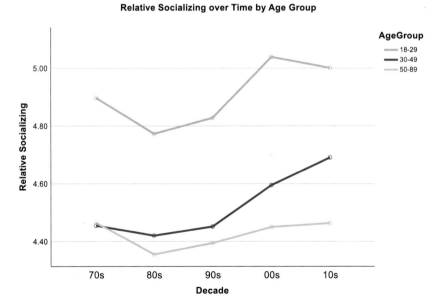

Fig. 4.7 Within age groups relative socializing declined then increased over time

1980s, and then there was a seemingly immediate reversal. The path upward since the 1990s is well-observed and significant. Young adult Americans have recently been spending social evenings with their relatives an average of "once or twice a week." The other age groups, of course, have been doing so less often than the youngsters, but more often than ever over the last some fifty years.[8]

These two figures clash with many reports from popular culture. Google searches for "loneliness" and "social isolation" in America yield myriad hits with labels like "crisis" and "epidemic." Some of this has been occasioned by the COVID-19 pandemic, of course, but Robert Putnam's famous bestseller *Bowling Alone* asserting "The collapse of American community" is over twenty years old. The author gives public speeches entitled "Is American Society Falling Apart?" Most of the attendees think they know the answer: yes.

So far, this chapter has offered an empirical rebuttal regarding friends and relatives. The neighboring data makes the opposite case. Figure 4.8 shows neighbor socializing plummeting through the 1990s, then

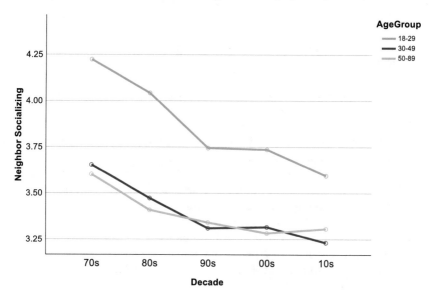

Fig. 4.8 Within age groups neighbor socializing has declined over time

apparently bottoming-out in the last two decades. This is true for all age groups, but especially so for young Americans who used to see their neighbors over "several times a month."[9] Not any more.

The present volume will not be caught up in any unitary narratives about the state of America. Such stories are always simpler than the reality. Our focus is on the sources of happiness and its accompaniments. Prominent among the latter are marriages, jobs, network relations—social structures, in other words. Some are waxing, some are waning, but all of them are relevant to personal well-being. Even this statement, though, is too simple. Findings about the state of happiness in America are exhilarating due to the power of GSS generalization, but they can be too sweeping. There are data-based indications that the pursuit of happiness has been creating great divides in American life, a matter to be addressed in Chap. 5.

In Their Own Words

Recall that when the qualitative sample was asked what are the "major factors in your life that make you happy," a common answer was being with "family and friends." It is telling that they offered this response unprompted, but the following question zeros in on those interactions:

> How has socializing with your friends and family contributed to your happiness?

Some respondents are decidedly not social butterflies. Edward, a disabled white male, simply says, "I am not that social of a person." A divorced white female in Duluth, Minnesota, replies, "I don't have a social life. I take care of children." A retired Asian male from Hawaii says that, "I am just lonely and I don't socialize with anyone."

Loneliness is a media theme mentioned above, and it appeared here with a twist. Jacob, a white salesman from San Jose offers, "It is nice just to have people around to avoid loneliness. Loneliness is the driving force of unhappiness …" A retired widow from Port Orchard, California, agrees: "Just having company around makes you happier; just them being around helps with the loneliness and that makes you happy." Most respondents do not appear to be lonely, and the twist is these folks know—and utilize—the social antidote.

Without using the term, a number of respondents are buoyed up by social support. A married engineer from Wisconsin says, "We have had good interaction with friends and associates and for the most part it has been very positive. We ... are there for each other in the death of friends and family ..." Help in coping with life's difficulties is a motif. According to Stacy from Albuquerque, "When you spent time with other people, you realize you are part of something; friends and family want to hang out with you and they share the same troubles." Steve, in law enforcement in California, gets right to the point: "Everyone is supportive of each other and when we have problems, we can talk and sort them out."

A couple of respondents noted the negative effects of socializing being shut off. Michael, a 34-year-old white high school teacher, feels the loss when the school year is over: "It is a big deal. It's not good when everyone is at work and I am at home during the summer. Just being with someone is a big deal." Marybeth, another teacher from Bristol, Florida also felt the loss during the pandemic: "After the 2020 shutdown ... not being able to get together and spend time and then getting back makes me value and appreciate it more."

But most people just extol the simple pleasures of being around friends and family. Marlyss, an 88-year-old Native American, puts it this way: "When we are together, we play cards and other kinds of games, talk and just enjoy each other." An 18-year-old Holly of Lansing, Michigan, says, "Every time I get to socialize or go to some sort of event with those I love it significantly improves my happiness."

NOTES

1. For the main effect of friend socializing, $F = 12.698$, $p < 0.001$; for the interaction effect of friend socializing-marital status, $F - 4.289$, $p < 0.001$.
2. In the four variable ANOVA not shown, the friend socializing-marital status-decade effect is $F = 1.047$, $p = $ n.s.
3. See Brian J. Jones, *Social Capital in American Life*, op. cit., 40.
4. For the main effect of relative socializing, $F = 18.549$, $p < 0.001$; for the interaction effect, $F = 2.311$, $p = 0.031$.
5. For the main effect of neighbor socializing, $F = 15.164$, $p < 0.001$; for the interaction effect, $F = 3.673$, $p = 0.001$.
6. For the main effect of decade, $F = 8.734$, $p < 0.001$.

7. For the main effect of decade, $F = 18.512$, $p < 0.001$; for the interaction effect of age-decade, $F = 5.342$, $p < 0.001$.
8. For the main effect of decade, $F = 20.125$, $p < 0.001$; for the interaction effect of age-decade, $F = 2.787$, $p = 0.004$.
9. For the main effect of decade, $F = 50.779$, $p < 0.001$; for the interaction effect of age-decade, $F = 2.937$, $p = 0.003$.

REFERENCE

Jones, Brian J., *Social Capital in American Life* (Palgrave Macmillan, 2019).

CHAPTER 5

"E PLURIBUS DUO": Education

Abstract Education level—specifically, college vs. non-college—has become a dividing line in our national life. Americans with a college degree are happier in their marriages, more satisfied with their jobs and happier overall. Over time marriage has declined much more rapidly among non-college Americans, and a college degree has become more strongly related to upper class position.

Keywords College vs. non-college

Few things in American life are more revered than education. It is the golden door, the key to movin' on up, the path to pulling up one's bootstraps on the ladder of success. It is the antidote to societal ills, the proposed panacea for poverty, drugs, crime, and a myriad of other social problems. More education cliches are available, but their multiplicity proves how we prize it.

Speaking of American things, our national motto is e pluribus unum—from the many, one. Despite our widely-shared reverence for schooling, there is emerging evidence that it can be a source of division. Cable news carries daily stories about political conflicts opposing Americans at different education levels. A previous book by this author entitled *Social Capital in American Life* evidenced a widening education-based divide in social

B. J. Jones, *The Pursuit of Happiness in America*,
https://doi.org/10.1007/978-3-031-65607-1_5

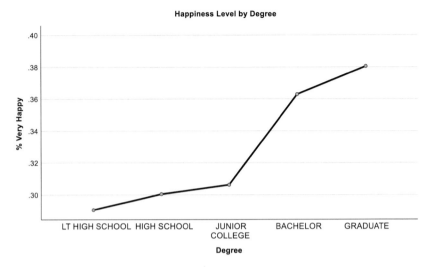

Fig. 5.1   Happiness level by degree

structures. The break point seems to be Americans who have been to college vs. those who have not. A simple duality.

But rather than prejudge the applicability of this cleavage to the happiness issue, consider Fig. 5.1. It displays education by degree versus the familiar happiness measure. The overall effect is statistically significant,[1] but observe the distinct break above junior college. Americans with a college degree have clearly elevated high happiness, and even more is added for those with graduate degrees. This informs the dichotomous measure in Fig. 5.2.[2]

DOES MONEY BUY HAPPINESS?

Many popular cliches link education to money, so they are unlinked in Fig. 5.3. The vertical spaces between the dots document the happiness effects of income, but the college dots are still higher than the non-college dots. The degree level effect of Fig. 5.2 has obviously been flattened out, but in a way this proves the cliches. Of course degrees are linked to income, that is ostensibly why people go to college. But even after the income-generating impact of college is netted out, there appears to be an additional "pure" effect of education.[3]

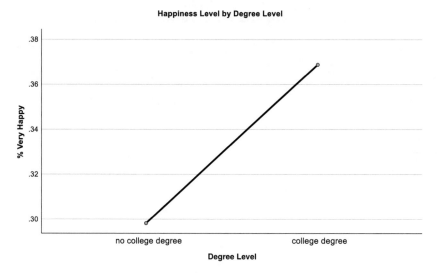

Fig. 5.2 Americans with a college degree are more likely to be very happy than those without a college degree

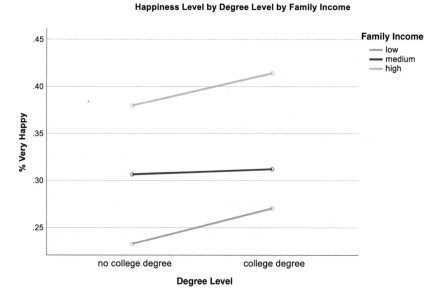

Fig. 5.3 Degree level and family income have independent effects on happiness

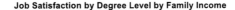

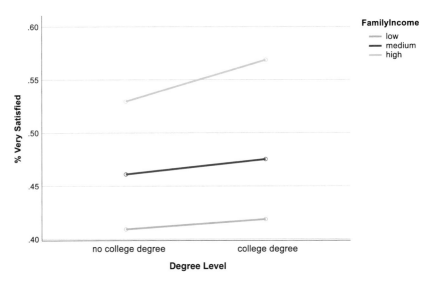

Fig. 5.4 Degree level and family income have independent effects on job satisfaction

Now that this is on the record, it will be useful to retrace our steps across the concomitants of happiness. Start with job satisfaction in Fig. 5.4, also incorporating money since salary is an important part of work. Degree level shows a moderate uptilt above college net of income, but, again, going to college is a path to better paying jobs.[4]

Marital happiness likewise requires an income control since family money is pooled. Figure 5.5 tells a more complex story. Start with the cluster of dots above college, all between 66% and 68% very happy with marriage. Income makes little difference over there, but a big difference above non-college. The tale this tells for the latter is that low income bottoms out marital happiness, middle income drops it a moderate amount, and high income has little additional effect.[5] Having been to college matters much to the marital happiness of American adults, especially the poorer ones.

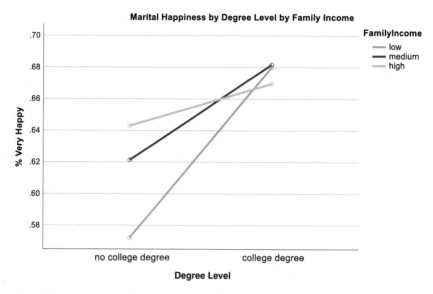

Fig. 5.5 Degree level has a stronger effect on marital happiness for Americans with lower levels of family income

SCHOOLING AND SOCIAL STRUCTURES

The latter finding points the way to the time dimension. The dynamic drop-off of marriage has been paralleled by a dynamic increase in formal schooling. According to the GSS data, the 13.3% of Americans who had (at least) a college degree in the 1970s had climbed to 29.5% by the 2010s. Do these trends interrelate?

They do. Figure 5.6 at first glance is a cascade of dot averages representing percent married. This much is well established, but not the degree level difference. Across the decades, marriage dropped about 15% for college Americans. For non-college adults, the numbers fell from 67.5% to 39.4%, a stunning decrement of 28.1%. This differential decline means that college Americans are now *much* more likely to be married, and that gap has widened in every decade.[6] Such findings resonate with Brookings Institution senior fellow Isabel Sawhill's statement that, "family formation is a new fault line in the American class structure."[7]

This statement sets the stage for the well-known intersection of schooling and social class. Figure 5.7 looks at it a bit differently. Here, the

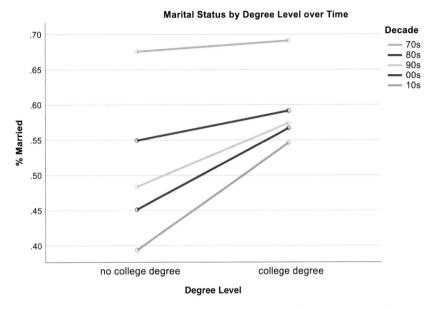

Fig. 5.6 Marriage has declined much more over time for Americans without a college degree

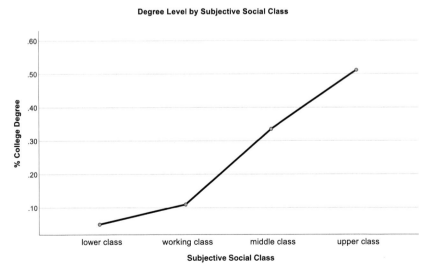

Fig. 5.7 The higher the subjective social class the more likely Americans are to have a college degree

percentage of Americans with (at least) a college degree is arrayed on the y-axis to display differences by subjective social class. This reveals yet another strikingly linear class effect strongly suggesting that tuition is the ticket to the American Dream.[8] Middle class adults, for instance, are *three times* as likely to have a degree in hand than working-class adults.

There are two complications. First, time again. Figure 5.8 replays the relationship across the decades and there are more differences. Of course, the dots rise over time with the spread of college, but note the slopes of the progressing lines. Decade to decade the percent with degrees has mounted up faster at each higher class.[9] This complication has a simple interpretation: there is more college than ever, *and* a degree matters more than ever up the rungs of the class ladder.[10]

The second complication involves gender.[11] As Fig. 5.9 clearly shows, the college-ification of America has proceeded faster for women than men. From a wide gap in degrees in the 1970s, the difference has virtually disappeared (less than 1%) in the most recent decade. Current statistics forecast a crossing of these lines in the immediate future. College enrollments are now 60% female versus 40% male, an inversion of the percentages at the start of the GSS.[12] Moreover, females have higher college completion rates and are outperforming males across the K-12 curriculum.[13]

The final site of the schooling separation is network socializing. Since Chap. 4 established major differences by relationship type, they are spotlighted here. Friending is much higher among degree holders in every decade (Fig. 5.10)[14]; relative visiting used to be much higher among non-college Americans, but the gap has closed considerably (Fig. 5.11)[15]; and despite the across-the-board downturn in neighboring, college Americans have done more of it in every decade (Fig. 5.12).[16]

At this empirical point, *e pluribus duo* no longer seems like a rhetorical flourish. By weight of evidence, colleged Americans are happier in general, happier with their marriages and happier with their jobs—all net of income. Uncolleged Americans, alternatively, have been exiting marriage at a greater rate and languishing at lower rungs of the class ladder. In terms of their social worlds, they are living very different lives. And, finally, the expansion of the college cohort promises to magnify these changes—especially for American women.

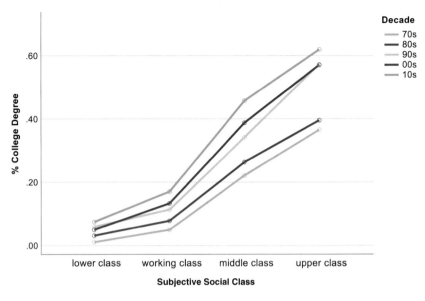

Fig. 5.8 Over time the likelihood that Americans with a higher subjective social class would have a college degree has increased

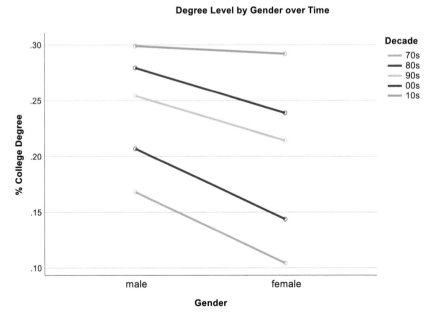

Fig. 5.9 Over time the gap in male vs. female college degrees has significantly closed

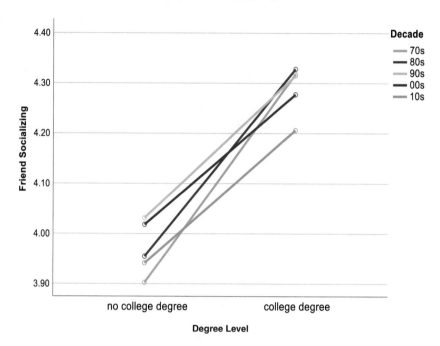

Fig. 5.10 Friend socializing has been higher among college vs. non-college Americans over time

In Their Own Words

The qualitative survey did not pose any direct questions about how respondents' educational backgrounds impacted their present happiness. For most, that background had been acquired decades earlier. Nevertheless, higher education did insert itself into several other answers.

Stacey, 35-year-old college graduate, lost her mother in college, but appears to have used that tragedy as inspiration: "After I got out of school, I was wanting to change the world and now I know what I can do." There are some folks not so inspired. Statistical programmer Irene, "… regrets spending lots of money applying to med school when I didn't want to be

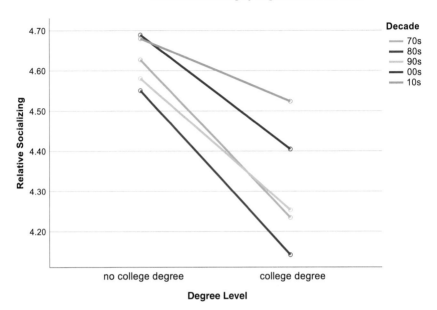

Fig. 5.11 Relative socializing used to be much higher among non-college than college Americans but the gap has closed over time

a doctor." Similarly, Emily, still a student, says, "The idea of knowing I will be in student debt for 20 to 30 years does not make me happy." Finally, a 69 year-old federal employee from Oakland receives vicarious satisfaction from the benefits of education: "My children are good to enjoy. They both have master's degrees and have jobs that pay them well …"

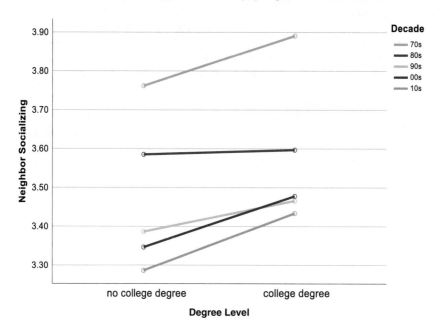

Fig. 5.12 Neighbor socializing has declined significantly among non-college and college Americans over time

NOTES

1. For the main effect of degree, $F = 61.463$, $p < 0.001$.
2. For the main effect of degree level, $F = 236.345$, $p < 0.001$.
3. For the main effect of income, $F = 254.931$, $p < 0.001$; for the main effect of degree level, $F = 21.649$, $p < 0.001$.
4. For the main effect of income, $F = 147.249$, $p < 0.001$; for the main effect of degree level, $F = 8.968$, $p = 0.003$.
5. For the main effect of degree level, $F = 34.763$, $p < 0.001$; for the main effect of income, $F = 2.079$, $p = $ n.s.; for the interaction effect, $F = 5.092$, $p = 0.006$.
6. For the main effect of decade, $F = 172.865$, $p < 0.001$; for the decade-degree level interaction, $F = 23.453$, $p < 0.001$.

7. Isabel Sawhill, *Generation Unbound: Drifting into Sex and Parenthood without Marriage* (Brookings Institution Press, 2014), 76.
8. For the main effect of subjective social class, $F = 2104.878$, $p < 0.001$.
9. For the main effect of decade, $F = 107.032$, $p < 0.001$; for the decade-class interaction effect, $F = 19.162$, $p < 0.001$.
10. Of course part of this dynamic is higher class, educated parents helping to secure their children's higher education. See, for example, Richard V. Reeves, *Dream Hoarders* (Brookings Institution Press, 2017).
11. For the decade-gender interaction effect, $F = 9.496$, $p < 0.001$.
12. See Scott Galloway, *Adrift: America in 100 Charts* (Transworld Publishers, 2022), 144–5.
13. Richard V. Reeves, *On Boys and Men* (Brookings Institution Press, 2022).
14. For the main effect of degree level, $F = 230.5091$ $p < 0.001$.
15. For the decade-degree level interaction effect, $F = 5.221$, $p < 0.001$.
16. For the main effect of degree level, $F = 14.241$, $p < 0.001$.

References

Galloway, Scott, *Adrift: America in 100 Charts* (Transworld Publishers, 2022).
Reeves, Richard V., *On Boys and Men* (Brookings Institution Press, 2022).
Sawhill, Isabel, *Generation Unbound: Drifting into Sex and Parenthood without Marriage* (Brookings Institution Press, 2014).

CHAPTER 6

Screen Time

Abstract Time spent on television and computer screens has been implicated as a negative force in American life. People who watch more TV are less happy, but the direction of causation is unclear. Time spent on email has been on the rise, but shows no significant relation to happiness. TV viewing time is positively associated with network socializing for all but older adults. Email hours are positively associated with network socializing across all age groups.

Keywords Televisivon hours • Email hours

> We have met the enemy,
> and he is us.
> - Pogo

There is some irony in opening this chapter with a quote from a comic strip character. *Pogo* was a satiric feature nationally syndicated in hundreds of U.S. newspapers from 1948 until 1975. The current generation will never have heard of it, which reflects generational shifts in mass media consumption. Newspapers have been disappearing and declining, especially after 1975. The internet, to put it mildly, is in its ascendancy. Television spans the generations.

B. J. Jones, *The Pursuit of Happiness in America*,
https://doi.org/10.1007/978-3-031-65607-1_6

Both of the latter forms of media have been the subject of dire predictions about American life. In *Bowling Alone*, Harvard political science professor Robert Putnam nominated television as a prime mover in the ostensible crash of social capital in the U.S. He also wondered, "will the Internet become predominantly a means of active, social communication or a means of passive, private entertainment? Will computer-mediated communication crowd out face-to-face ties?"[1] We wonder, too.

TELEVISION VIEWING

A reasonable place to begin is with how much time Americans have devoted to television according to the following GSS question:

On the average day, how many hours do you personally watch television?

Two things are apparent in Fig. 6.1. First, Americans invest considerable time in their TV screens. The national average across the board is just under three hours. Second, there is no discernible trend. Even the widest swing in the data (1978–1980) is well under half an hour, and the final dot average (2018) is only a few minutes away from the starting point (1975).

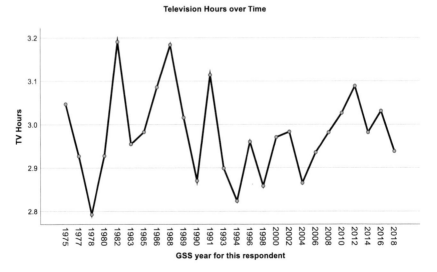

Fig. 6.1 Americans' average hours watching television over time

Does watching television have anything to do with personal happiness? The answer is yes. Figure 6.2 shows a clear decrease in percent very happy with increases in TV viewing level.[2] Folks who watch at least four hours a day are a full 9% less likely to check the highest happiness box than 0–1 hour viewers. But wait. This is another cross-sectional result with an alternative interpretation. That alternative is displayed in Fig. 6.3. Switching the axes produces a very similar effect line depicting very happy people watching less television.

So the TV-happiness connection can be read two ways. The next two chapters will engage causal direction by introducing panel data that open the time dimension. But some data-based observations can be offered here. First, the amount of television watched seems to depend on how busy people are. A simple life-cycle analysis in Fig. 6.4 depicts a major dip in the 30 s and 40 s when work and family are at peak demand, then a steady rise in hours viewed as leisure time presents itself. This suggests that television is a time-filler rather than a happiness-stealer, but more direct evidence is available from a different data source. John Robinson and his colleagues have performed a series of studies using time diaries, in which people record what they are actually doing during the hours of the day.[3] One study using this approach took temporality into account:

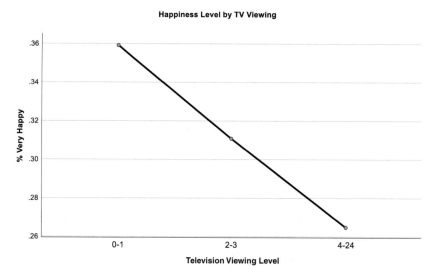

Fig. 6.2 Americans who watch more TV are less likely to be very happy

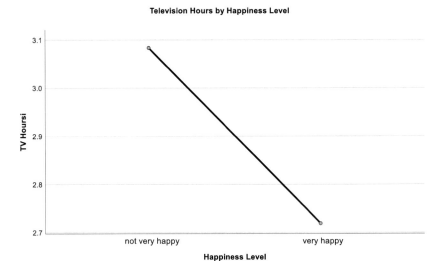

Fig. 6.3   Americans who are very happy watch less TV than the not very happy

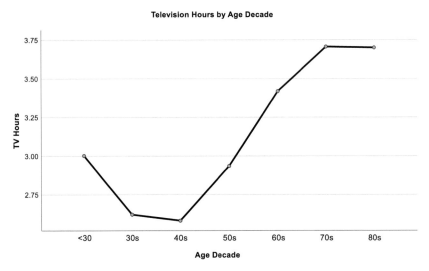

Fig. 6.4   Americans in busier work and family decades watch less TV

Respondents reported time spent watching TV as well as positive affect for eight consecutive days. Results of multilevel modeling analyses showed that duration of TV watching on the previous day did not significantly predict changes in positive affect on the next day. However, *positive affect on the previous day predicted decreases in duration of TV watching the following day* (emphasis added).[4]

Positive affect would seem to be more a matter of mood than overall happiness, but at first glance (subject to the expanded view of Chap. 8), the evidence that television viewing leads to unhappiness is tenuous at best.

EMAIL USE

Again, we begin with an assessment of screen time. The GSS item initiated in 2020 is the following:

About how many hours per week do you spend sending and answering email?

Figure 6.5 shows the steady growth of this contemporary form of interpersonal communication. By 2018 the national average had grown to over

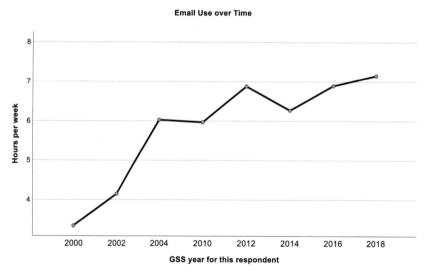

Fig. 6.5 Hours Americans spend on email have increased over time

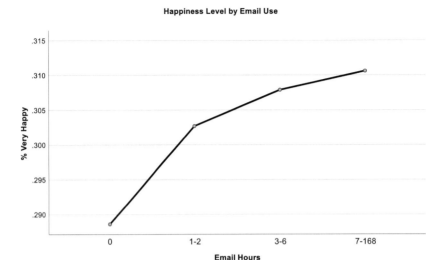

Fig. 6.6   The association between email hours and happiness is positive but not statistically significant

an hour a day per American with many, of course, spending much more time. Does more email impact happiness? According to Fig. 6.6, not in any meaningful way. The apparent increase spans only about one-tenth of one percent of high happiness, clearly not significant.[5] On the other hand, these data give rebuttal to a spate of recent articles declaring that "Email is making us miserable."

Consider for a moment what lies behind these two screens. Television is a form of entertainment which can be consumed in solitary or social fashion. Email, as it is phrased above, is a "form of interpersonal communication." Whatever their linkages to personal happiness, both types of electronic media have implicated linkages to everyday social interaction.

SCREEN TIME AND SOCIALIZING

In response to the GSS question, quite a few respondents say that they "personally watch television" 24 hours a day. This raises the specter of lonely Americans with only their boob tubes for company. Notions that television is an instrument of isolation are dispelled by Fig. 6.7. It features network socializing—the composite scale adding up social evenings spent

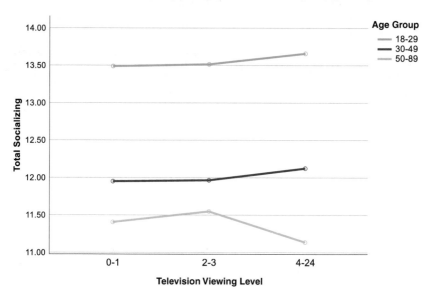

Fig. 6.7   TV viewing is positively associated with network socializing for 18–29 and 30–49 but not for 50–89 age groups

with friends, relatives, and neighbors. Be reminded that these are in-person interactions, not Facebook encounters. Also be reminded that age exerts such a salient suppressive effect on going out that it must be included in the analyses. So, TV viewing appears to exert very mild effects on network socializing. For 18- to 29-year-olds and 30- to 49-year-olds it is actually mildly positive; for Americans 50 and older, it is comparably negative. Moreover, decade-by-decade analyses (not shown) demonstrate that this is a persistent pattern.[6] Clearly, we are not a nation of TV-addicted hermits.

But is electronic communication driving out face-to-face communication? Not according to Fig. 6.8. In fact, more hours emailing means more "social evenings" for all three age groups, but especially so for middle age and older adults.[7]

It is worth reflecting on these results from a common sense perspective. TV viewing can be an escape, but it also can be a social occasion. Specific program content is not available here, but *The Bachelor, Real Housewives*

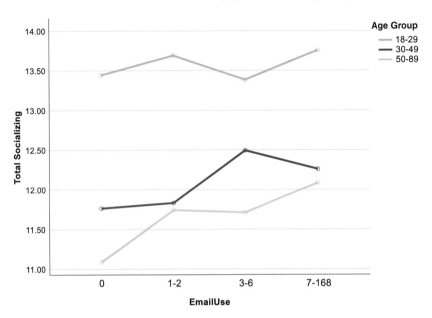

Fig. 6.8 Email use is positively associated with network socializing for all age groups

and *Game of Thrones* watch parties are real things. Who watches the Superbowl alone? And *why* do people email each other? One obvious reason is to set things up. Arranging a lunch date or movie night is conveniently done by email on laptop, tablet or telephone. Speaking of the latter, the GSS through the end of the last decade does not offer sufficient data to analyze texting or the impact of social media through Facebook (meta), Twitter (x) or Instagram. The Pew Research Center has conducted a series of studies across these media such as the Personal Networks and Community Survey which generally concur with the pro-social results reported here.[8]

At this point, there is not even a prima facie case to be made that screen time is socially destructive "me time." Claims that electronic hours are eroding happiness are unproven and, frankly, counterintuitive. Both TV and email are clearly compatible with active social lives. Pogo's newspaper-mediated wisdom does not seem applicable to more modern means of communication.

In Their Own Words

Screen time is another topic not specifically interrogated in the qualitative questionnaire. Nevertheless, television programming popped up as a source of happiness. Among the things that make student Emily happy are, "Netflix, family and friends." An unmarried, biracial woman from Baltimore offers, "I am a big Star Trek fan and that makes me happy." Aimee, 25-year-old bookstore employee, says, "The major factors in my life that make me happy are my best friend and my favorite show called Camp Camp." These idiosyncratic answers are not substantive enough to offer proof on the TV-happiness causal direction except in a single case. Daniel, a retired widower from Honolulu reports that his health is deteriorating and, "…I can't do anything at all except watch TV."

No respondent volunteered an opinion about time spent on email, but some computer screen issues did appear. "Too much social media for kids" contributes to making an unemployed, divorced Duluth, Minnesota woman less happy. Travis, a disabled 40-year-old from Panorama City, South Carolina, says, "The downside of the internet is that you cannot have any connection with anyone." Several respondents beg to differ. Patrick, a Dallas 63-year-old, says one reason he is happy is because, "I enjoy helping people online when they have questions about electronics." In response to the socializing-contributing-to happiness question, statistical programmer Irene says, "With friends, it is nice having someone to play video games with." Also referencing the screen-social connection, Bill the manufacturing worker/comedian offers this: "The social network thing (Facebook) is the stupidest thing ever, but it brought us (he and his wife) together."

Notes

1. Robert D. Putnam, *Bowling Alone: The Collapse and Revival of American Community* (Simon & Schuster, 2000).
2. For the main effect of happiness level, $F = 191.367$, $p < 0.001$.
3. See John P. Robinson and Steven Martin, "Of Time and Television," *Annals of the American Academy of Political and Social Science* (Vol. 625, 2009), 82.
4. Deniz Bayraktaroglu, Gul Gunaydin, Emre Selcuk, and Anthony D. Ong, "A Daily Diary Investigation of the Link Between Television Watching and Positive Affect," *Journal of Happiness Studies* (Vol. 20, 2018), 1099.
5. For the main effect of email use, $F = 1.065$, p = n.s.

6. For the TV viewing-age interaction effect, $F = 11.039$, $p \leq 0.001$. For the TV viewing-age decade interaction effect, $F = 0.878$, $p =$ n.s.
7. For the email use-age interaction effect, $F = 3.527$, $p < 0.001$.
8. For example, "People's use of the mobile phone and internet is associated with larger and more diverse discussion networks." Pew Research Center, "Social Isolation and New Technology," (Nov. 4, 2009), 1.

REFERENCES

Bayraktaroglu, Deniz, Gul Gunaydin, Emre Selcuk, and Anthony D. Ong, "A Daily Diary Investigation of the Link between Television Watching and Positive Affect," *Journal of Happiness Studies*, (Vol. 20, 2018), 1089–1101.

Putnam, Robert D., *Bowling Alone: The Collapse and Revival of American Community* (Simon & Schuster, 2000).

Robinson, John P., and Steven Martin, "Of Time and Television," *Annals of the American Academy of Political and Social Science* (Vol. 625, 2009). 74–86.

CHAPTER 7

Lost Causes

Abstract Panel studies facilitate the search for causal direction by re-interviewing respondents over time. In this chapter, the 2006–2008 GSS panel is highlighted. The multivariate analyses favor the conclusion that earlier marriage favors later happiness rather than previous happiness level leading to later marriage. Modeling the causal direction of the network socializing—happiness correlation is hampered by very little change in 2006–2008 socializing. However, 2006 socializing is significantly positively associated with 2008 happiness for older and married Americans.

Keywords Correlation vs. causation

A quick flip-thvrough of this book reveals a profusion of rising effect lines, telltales of powerful statistical associations. Perhaps the most singular is the connection of marriage to personal happiness. Despite its formidable strength, the methodological chapter-and-verse is to not confuse such *correlations* with *causation*. It is time for a deeper probe. Perhaps lost causes can be found, or at least better targeted.

Better addressing cause and effect is a major reason that the GSS has conducted a series of panel studies in which the same respondents are re-interviewed over time. This opens the door of temporality to determine what happens to a given factor *after* some other factor, an inference that

B. J. Jones, *The Pursuit of Happiness in America*,
https://doi.org/10.1007/978-3-031-65607-1_7

cannot be drawn if both factors are measured simultaneously. The latter limitation of cross-sectional studies is why panels are considered a pathway to causality in the social sciences.[1]

In addition to its standard longitudinal, cross-sectional data, the GSS has administered several panels. The most recent covered 2016–2018–2020. This was not a full panel because 2016 and 2018 respondents were re-interviewed only once, in 2020. That year is notable because of the onset of COVID-19, an event producing such unique societal changes (including a bottoming-out of personal happiness) that it will be spotlighted in Chap. 8. The first GSS panel covered 2006–2008–2010. Again, the latter year was unique since it occurred on the heels of the Great Recession and produced by far the lowest happiness profile over the entire 1972–2018 time span. So, the present chapter will focus on the 2006–2008 re-interviews as a more typical timeline.[2]

Marriage and Happiness

Begin with the analytical conclusions from Chap. 3:

> Across the five decades, marriage roughly doubles the chance of being very happy, 40.4% to 21.1% … This effect exists for males and females, for blacks and whites, for young and old … indeed, for every variable the author has conceived of and tested.

The robustness of the marriage-happiness effect across the myriad of control variables is persuasive—but circumstantial—evidence. It still allows reasonable doubts about marriage's causal status.

Figure 7.1 commences evaluating the evidence by examining the happiness impact of marriage in 2006 two years later. The familiar effect line breaks down into 35.6% very happy for those married before 2008 compared to 22.8% for the previously unmarried.[3] Since future happiness cannot predict past marriage, this is exhibit A in the argument for the pro-marriage effect.

There are, however, two complications. First, change in marital status may have intervened between 2006 and 2008; unmarried folks could have gotten hitched, and marriages could have dissolved. Figure 7.2 takes this directly into account. The red line traces the effect of 2008 marriage upon 2008 happiness for those married in 2006; the blue line does the same for the previously unmarried. The result is uncomplicated. Both respondents

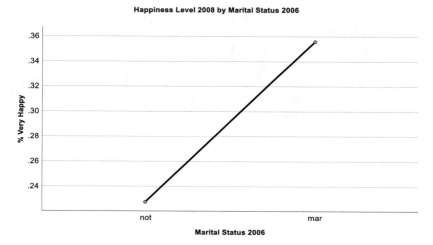

Fig. 7.1   Panel respondents married in 2006 were more likely to be very happy in 2008 than those previously unmarried

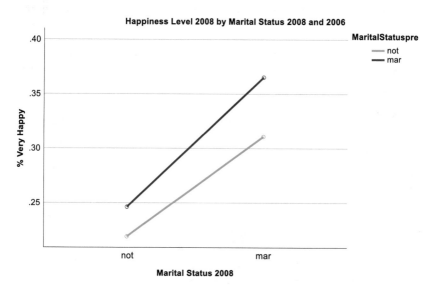

Fig. 7.2   Panel respondents were more likely to be very happy if married in 2008 whether they were married or unmarried in 2006

who were and were not in prior marriages are significantly happier if currently married in 2008.[4]

Complication number two concerns prior happiness levels. The possibility that the correlation may be caused by happier folks getting married receives no support here. In Fig. 7.3 the Y-axis is percent married in 2008. Note that singles in 2006 who were very happy actually are a little *less* likely to have gotten married by 2008 (the right blue dot is 7.7% compared to 10.3% for the left blue dot).

Figure 7.4 incorporates both complications to arrive at a simple conclusion. Panel 7.4a displays 2008 happiness levels for respondents who were not very happy in 2006. There is little change for those already married, but the newly married unhappies soar far above the still unmarried. At least as impressive is Panel 7.4b displaying those already very happy in 2006. *Both* respondents who were and were not married before get significantly happier if married in 2008.[5] Marriage seems to magnify happiness even among the already very happy.

Previous researchers have scrutinized the marriage-happiness connection and reached largely confirmatory conclusions. A recent report in the

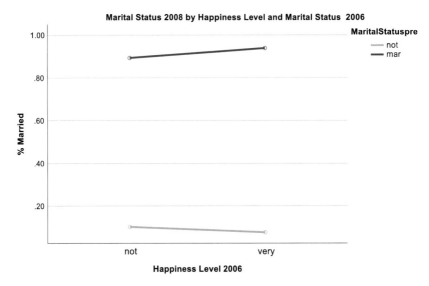

Fig. 7.3 Panel respondents who were very happy and unmarried in 2006 were not more likely to be married in 2008

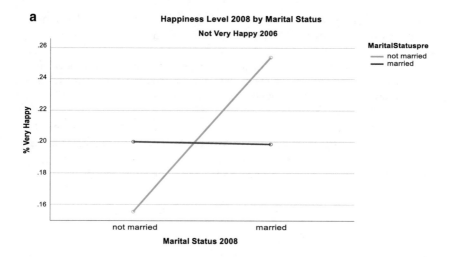

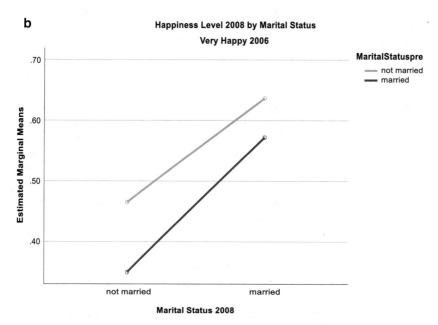

Fig. 7.4 **a** Panel respondents who were not very happy and unmarried in 2006 were more likely to be very happy if married in 2008. **b** Panel respondents who were very happy in 2006 were more likely to be very happy if married in 2008 regardless of previous marital status

Journal of Happiness Studies analyzed data from the U.S., the United Kingdom and Germany. Chapman and Guven observe that,

> The relationship between marriage and happiness has been studied widely in a range of social science disciplines and there is a comfortable consensus that marriage has a positive and enduring influence on well-being.[6]

Moreover, one conclusion from their analyses is definitive: "A strong link from happiness to marriage does not exist."[7] The value-added from the present analysis—that is, Fig. 7.4—is that even if it *did* exist, marriage seems to further enhance happiness for happy and unhappy alike.

Network Socializing and Happiness

Chapter 3 also tabled the causality question with regard to the socializing-happiness connection documented here and elsewhere. Ruut Veenhoven, founder of *The Journal of Happiness Studies*, thinks the most plausible model is a virtuous cycle in which interaction produces happiness *and* happiness gives rise to further interaction.[8] In a book chapter entitled, "Happiness and Sociability in a Nonrecursive Model," Ming-Chang Tsai observes, "Research that has explored the reverse causal direction (i.e., happiness leading to interaction), however, is scant in the literature." A major reason is the scarcity of panel studies that allow such exploration.[9]

The present project has such rare data at hand. The most elegant test of a reciprocal relationship involves the creation of change measures across the 2006–2008 interim. Specifically, compute happiness change and socializing change, then determine how they are interconnected. The attempt to do so encountered a problem that is also an empirical finding: there is precious little change in people's social lives over time. Be reminded that network socializing is a scale totaling social evenings spent with friends plus relatives plus neighbors, each scored one (about once a year) through six (almost every day). So: in an eighteen point index, the average change from 2006 to 2008 was -0.18, well less than a single scale point; the median change was zero. Clearly, Americans' social lives are, well, social structures.

Given the fact that network socializing is a virtual constant, the best approach is to simply project 2006 socializing upon future—that is, 2008—happiness levels. Figure 7.5 does so, and the effect is in the expected direction, but not quite statistically significant.[10] Despite the

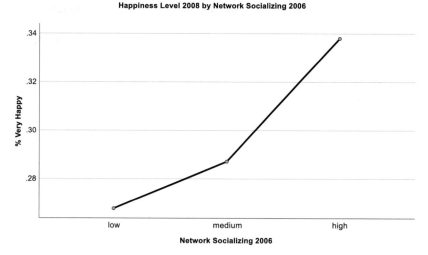

Fig. 7.5 Network socializing in 2006 was positively but not significantly associated with happiness in 2008

constancy of socializing, happiness does change over time so a stricter test is to put both happiness levels in play. Figure 7.6 again shows the expected upturn in percent very happy 2008 for both happiness levels in 2006, and again the socializing effect approaches but does not attain significance.[11]

Two data lessons that have been learned must now enter the analysis. The first concerns age. Figure 7.7 deepens the earlier find that network socializing is especially potent for older Americans. The mixed results for 18- to 29-year-olds and 30- to 49-year-olds resolves into a powerful upsweep in subsequent happiness for those over 50.[12] Chapter 4 documented that "socializing magnifies the pro-happiness effect of marriage." Figure 7.8 extends this with the time dimension. Folks already married in 2006 show a much greater happiness response to network socializing in 2008.[13]

In Their Own Words

An alternative approach to the causality question is to just ask people about changes in their happiness. The following set of interview items did just that:

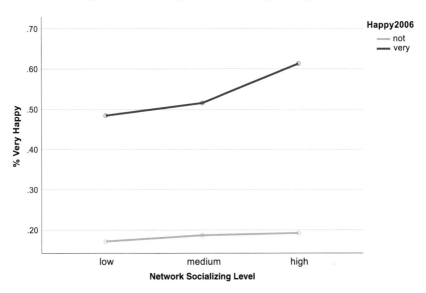

Fig. 7.6 Network socializing in 2006 was positively but not significantly associated with happiness in 2008 for panel members both very and not very happy in 2006

> Has your level of happiness changed over time? For example, would you say you are more or less happy than a year ago?
> More
> Less
> The same
>
> How about compared to 10 years ago?
> More
> Less
> The same

> What would you say are some of the *main reasons* your level of happiness has changed over the years? (emphasis added)

Judging by the qualitative data, happiness is quite a dynamic state. Only five respondents remained "the same" over both the one-year and ten-year interims. More folks increased than decreased their happiness levels during each time period, but quite a few moved in both directions. Statistical

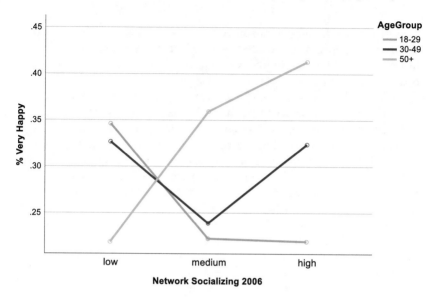

Fig. 7.7 Network socializing in 2006 was positively and significantly associated with happiness for 50–89 year olds in 2008

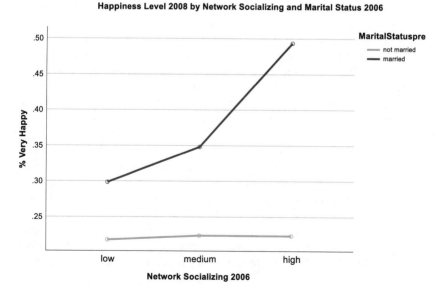

Fig. 7.8 Network socializing had a more powerful positive effect on happiness in 2008 for panel members married vs. unmarried in 2006

generalizations are not appropriate for this sample, but the dynamism apparent here speaks to the advisability of the multivariate analyses earlier in this chapter. Untangling causes requires measuring happiness level at dual time points due to its changeability.

Offering the "main reasons" for change means respondents are attributing causality. A number of them cited inner resources. Stacie, 52-year-old, reports she is happier because she acquired "wisdom as I age." Similarly (but not in spelling), Stacy the 35-year-old violin shop worker says, "I have grown up and I have a lot more tools in my toolbox." For some, the happiness tool is their faith. Patrick of Dallas, Texas, reports this main reason: "It is my faith in Christ. It has served to improve my happiness and my wisdom has had a great effect."

Using other terms, several respondents describe "economic position" from Chap. 3 as a happiness changer. Biracial social worker Summer blames "Financial and economic hardships" for her waning happiness. From the other side Bill, who works in manufacturing says, "I am living the American Dream. I work and get money and everything just pans out." For some, that dream is the end of work. A very happy white female reports, "I have quite a bit of reduced stress because I retired. I loved my work, but it was stressful."

A number of interviewees indicate that the prime mover of their happiness has been family life—for good and ill. Several like "b," a biracial Baltimorean woman, have family members who have passed to ill effect: "I lost my grandmother and that was a big blow because that was my support system." A 911 operator from Conyers, Georgia says that, "The happy things are my family and striving to do better and that makes me happier." Rene, a private investigator on capital murder cases, gives a few reasons, but she concludes with, "Relief that my kids are good people is quite beautiful."

Family life of course overlaps with the "network socializing" analyses undertaken above, but the factor that emerged most clearly here is marriage. It was mentioned most often as a main reason for happiness change and described in a causal fashion. Again, there is both negative and positive. Jill, a legal assistant from Greensboro, North Carolina, has a husband who suffered a "traumatic brain injury due to a motorcycle accident" that makes her "feel more like a caregiver than a spouse." An 80-year-old widow in Hughson, Nevada, reports that she is not too happy and that, "I don't have my husband here, he was the love of my life." The implication, of course, is that her husband was a source of happiness before the tragedy. A few respondents speak of a kind of happiness roller coaster as they moved from a bad to a good partner. So says Michael, a Native American teacher in Elkins, New York: "Getting divorced from someone who was hard to live with made it harder in life and having someone now who cares for me and appreciates me makes it easier in life." For TVM, a Philadelphia hair stylist, cause-and-effect is obvious: "I got married and it has been fantastic ever since."

NOTES

1. See Steven E. Finkel, *Causal Analysis with Panel Data* (Sage Publications, 2011).
2. For 2006, $n = 4510$. For 2008, $n = 1536$. The latter is the re-interview total.
3. For the main effect of 2006 marriage, $F = 30.960$, $p < 0.001$.
4. For the main effect of 2008 marriage, $F = 6.929$, $p < 0.001$.
5. For the main effect of 2008 marriage, $F = 6.946$, $p < 0.001$.
6. Bruce Chapman and Cahit Guven, "Revisiting the Relationship between Marriage and Wellbeing: Does Marriage Quality Matter?" *Journal of Happiness Studies* (Vol. 17, 2016), 533–534.
7. Ibid., 533.
8. Ruut Veenhoven, "Capability and Happiness: Conceptual Differences and Reality Links," *Journal of Socio-Economics* (Vol. 39, 2010), 349.
9. Ming-Chang Tsai, "Happiness and Sociability in a Nonrecursive Model: The US and Taiwan Compared" in *A Life Devoted to the Quality of Life*, edited by Filomena Maggino (Springer Cham, 2016), 300.
10. For the main effect of network socializing, $F = 2.165$, $p = 0.115$. Repeating the analysis for 2008 network socializing produces nearly identical results.
11. For the main effect of network socializing, $F = 2.411$, $p = 0.090$.
12. For the interaction effect of network socializing and age, $F = 3.701$, $p < 0.005$.
13. For the interaction effect of network socializing and marital status, $F = 4.057$, $p = 0.018$.

REFERENCES

Chapman, Bruce, and Cahit Guven, "Revisiting the Relationship between Marriage and Wellbeing: Does Marriage Quality Matter?" *Journal of Happiness Studies* (Vol. 17, 2016), 533–546.

Finkel, Steven E., *Causal Analysis with Panel Data* (Sage Publications, 2011).

Tsai, Ming-Chang, "Happiness and Sociability in a Nonrecursive Model: The US and Taiwan Compared" in *A Life Devoted to the Quality of Life*, edited by Filomena Maggino (Springer Cham, 2016), 297–314.

Veenhoven, Ruut, "Capability and Happiness: Conceptual Differences and Reality Links," *Journal of Socio-Economics* (Vol. 39, 2010), 344–350.

CHAPTER 8

Happiness Dynamics in the Age of Covid-19

Abstract This final chapter uses a panel sample spanning 2018 and the onset of Covid-19 in 2020. Over this interim, the distribution of happiness in America shifted significantly downward. The Covid-19 concern level was significantly associated with 2020 happiness, as well as a downward drop in happiness over 2018–2020. Network socializing also dropped but not significantly. Email use declined somewhat as television viewing rose. In 2020, the association of social class-happiness weakened considerably, and socializing-happiness was not statistically significant. The marriage effect on happiness remained clear and significant in the midst of Covid-19.

Keywords Covid-19 concern levels

Covid-19 has been a sociological singularity. It is a useful analogy. The counterpart of Einstein's idea of a space-time altering force is that of a pandemic shaking society to its roots. But it is time to transcend analogies.

The General Social Survey conducted an unusual panel study spanning 2016–2018–2020.[1] To be clear, respondents were not interviewed at all three time points. The year 2016 interviewees were reinterviewed only once in 2020, and the same for 2018 interviewees. But its most, well, singular feature concerned the timing of the 2020 survey. On March 11,

B. J. Jones, *The Pursuit of Happiness in America*, https://doi.org/10.1007/978-3-031-65607-1_8

2020, the World Health Organization declared Covid-19 a pandemic. Two days later the U.S. declared a national emergency and issued distancing guidelines that rendered the standard GSS personal interviews impossible. This delayed administration of the surveys until August 24 to September 26 of 2020, and necessitated web and phone data collection from the respondents personally interviewed in 2018.

Things Changed

This section title seems almost ironic. The Covid-19 phenomenon had many and varied impacts generating too massive of a literature to summarize here. Begin, therefore, with a simple focus on happiness in America. Figure 8.1 redeploys the original happiness item with all three responses. "Not very" and "pretty" happy are uncombined from the usual dichotomy versus "very" happy. The respective percentages are 14.3, 55.8, and 29.9—putting 2018 very much in line with typical GSS responses. Note the obvious shift in Fig. 8.2. That is the frequency distribution for 2020 as Covid-19 sets in. The high and low ends of happiness have, in effect, switched with "not very" at 29.2% and "very" at 18.4%.

The re-engineered GSS for 2020 included a brand new question:

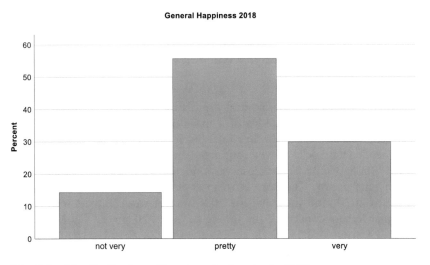

Fig. 8.1 The distribution of happiness in America in 2018

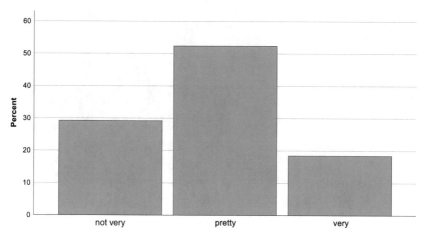

Fig. 8.2   The distribution of happiness in America in 2020

How concerned are you, if at all, about the corona virus or Covid-19 outbreak?

Figure 8.3 clearly shows concern clustered at the high levels with "very concerned" (30.7%) barely exceeding "extremely concerned" (26.7%.). So, high happiness fell to an unprecedented degree and a new source of stress soared to the nth degree. A connection seems likely.

For maximum transparency testing this connection, crosstabulation is the method of choice. Table 8.1 displays a drop in the "very happy" column at right as Covid-19 concern rises. More striking yet is the rise in the "not very" column from more pandemic stress; a full 37.8% of folks who are "extremely concerned" about the virus are "not too happy." This table contains a statistically significant connection,[2] and it suggests an even more focused approach. The magnification is turned up by creating a happiness change measure spanning 2018–2020.[3] The right-hand column of Table 8.2 displays the percent who got happier during this interim, which drops like a stone with greater concern. The opposite trend is manifest at left where dropping happiness nearly doubles from "not at all" (23.4%) to "extremely" (43.5%) concerned. This is, (1) a statistically significant result,[4] and (2) a key instance in which panel data can offer sharper insights into "Happiness Dynamics."

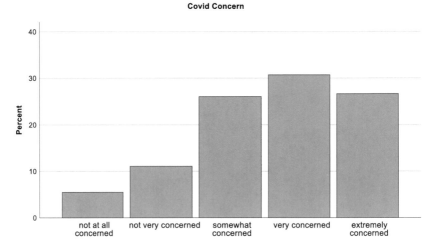

Fig. 8.3   Levels of concern about Covid-19 in 2020

Table 8.1   Happiness by Covid concern

	Not very	*Pretty*	*Very*
Wrycovz			
Not at all concerned	24	53	21
	24.5%	54.1%	21.4%
Not very concerned	49	103	44
	25.0%	52.6%	22.4%
Somewhat concerned	109	264	89
	23.6%	57.1%	19.3%
Very concerned	153	292	100
	28.1%	53.6%	18.3%
Extremely concerned	179	224	70
	37.8%	47.4%	14.8%

Things Stayed the Same

"Covid changed everything" has become a cultural cliché. Like most clichés, it is both true and false. The section immediately above testifies to its truth; other changes appear to have been exaggerated.

The present analysis has resorted to panel data to focus on change. That expectation looms even larger here given the events of 2020. Be reminded that Chap. 7 found remarkably tiny shifts in network socializing over

Table 8.2 Happiness change by Covid concern

	Down	*Same*	*Up*
Not at all concerned			
Count	15	33	16
	23.4%	51.6%	25.0%
Not very concerned			
Count	38	56	16
	34.5%	50.9%	14.5%
Somewhat concerned			
Count	85	127	35
	34.4%	51.4%	14.2%
Very concerned			
Count	85	177	30
	29.1%	60.6%	10.3%
Extremely concerned			
Count	117	131	21
	43.5%	48.7%	7.8%

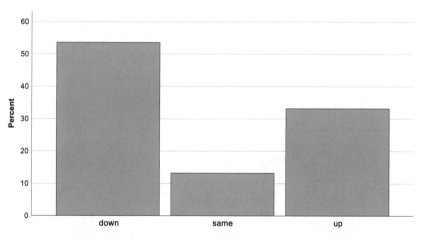

Network Socializing Change 2018-2020

Fig. 8.4 Network socializing change among panel respondents 2018–2020

2006–2008. Figure 8.4 displays evidence of such change for 2018–2020. Over half of respondents reduced their socializing over the interim as one would expect with social distancing. However, about a third of Americans actually *increased* their interaction, and the *degree* of "down" is pretty miniscule: -0.78, which is less than a single point on an 18 point scale. "Remarkably tiny" indeed.

Chapter 6 explored the link between "screen time" and socializing without panel-based change measures. Figure 8.5 offers such a measure for email hours which is surprisingly balanced. The actual numbers underlying the figure do show a decline of about an hour and a half a week—only about 13 minutes a day—and the median change is zero hours. For TV in Fig. 8.6 nearly half of the sample increase their screen time, certainly to be expected with folks staying home. How much of an increase? Well less than an hour a day, and again the median is zero.[5]

These relatively minor perturbations in everyday life highlight the hyperbole in "covid changed everything." They also preclude any meaningful analysis interrelating changes in socializing and screen time.

Social Structure Under Covid-19

In many ways Chap. 3 is the beating heart of this book. It featured the salient happiness social structures of class, marriage and network socializing. How have they functioned during the singular shock of Covid-19?

First up is subjective social class, which for five decades "demonstrated quasi-linear association with happiness". Figure 8.7 shows a very different

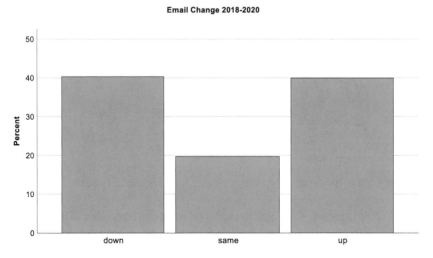

Fig. 8.5 Email hours change among panel respondents 2018–2020

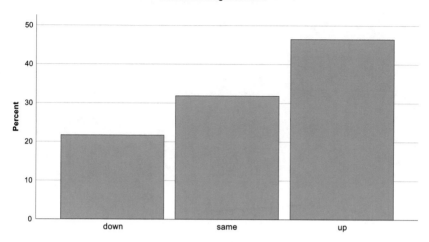

Fig. 8.6 TV viewing hours change among panel respondents 2018–2020

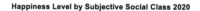
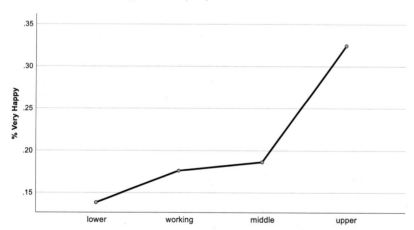

Fig. 8.7 The association between subjective social class and happiness weakened in 2020

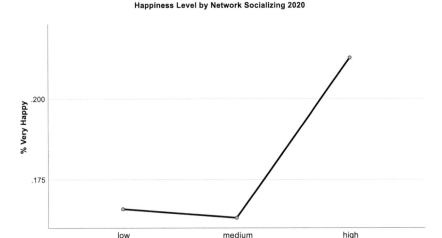

Fig. 8.8 The association between network socializing and happiness was positive but not significant in 2020

picture. Pre-2020, each higher class rung registered a gain in "very happy" of around ten percent. Here, the three left-hand classes collectively span barely five percent. The association is statistically significant,[6] but it is mainly driven by the soaring height of upper-class happiness.

As we have just seen, network socializing was very mildly suppressed during early Covid. How about its happiness impact? Figure 8.8 exhibits little change from low to medium social evenings spent, then a clear upsurge in percent very happy with high socializing. The effect is not quite statistically significant,[7] but Chap. 4 proved the necessity of taking marriage into account when framing the effects of socializing.

Marriage, of course, needs to be taken into account on its own. Figure 8.9 shows a pretty much unchanged relationship to happiness. Percent very happy more than doubles for married vs. unmarried Americans in 2020 (11.3% to 26.0%). As with all the figures in this section, high happiness is down but here the marriage effect remains robust.[8]

The dual effect of marriage and network socializing is featured in Fig. 8.10. Its display visually confirms two statistically significant relationships. The red dots looming above the blue are indicators that marriage magnifies happiness, and the dots peak at right indicating that network socializing does the

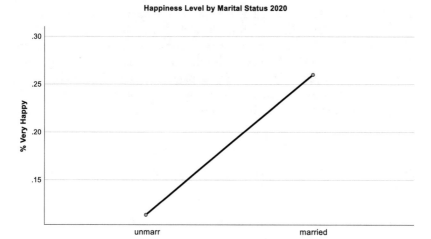

Fig. 8.9 The association between marriage and happiness was positive and significant in 2020

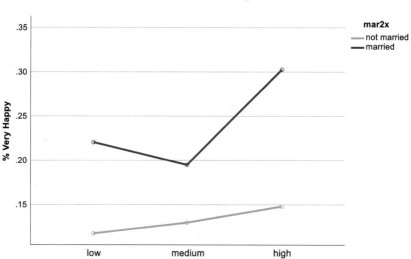

Fig. 8.10 Within both marital statuses, the association between network socializing and happiness was positive and significant in 2020

same.[9] So Covid-19 cast a pall across the land. Happiness plummeted, and Covid concern clearly had much to do with it. Despite seemingly obvious implications for stay-at-home electronic communication and entertainment—email and TV—the needle barely budged. The raw amount of a seemingly volatile use of time during a plague—face-to-face socializing—budged even less. And even with a national low tide in happiness, major social structures continued to buoy it up.

In Their Own Words

The final question in the qualitative survey asked respondents to identify their ultimate happiness cause:

> What single factor—an event, an experience or a person—has had the greatest effect on your level of happiness?

Of course, happiness has multiple causes in any complex life, but selecting the most potent factor is a very personal choice.

And, to that point, some select their own personality as the "single factor." Oft-quoted Stacie says, "I only rely on myself, so I will never be disappointed." A very happy female private investigator cites a singular personal insight: "Realizing that I wasn't just the passenger, I am in command."

A handful of folks give the credit to their religious beliefs and activities. For John, a retiree in Payson, New York, the single factor is, "My relationship with our father in heaven." Edward of Afton, Wyoming, "served two years as a missionary. I did things for other people rather than myself. It gave me a long-term sense of accomplishment."

Family and friends are common responses. Several select deaths and declining health of relatives as key negative events, but others disclose the simple joy of being with loved ones. An 81-year-old black woman in Pennsylvania picks, "My children. We have a good relationship and (they) genuinely love me and have my best interests at heart … and being there when you need them." Salesman Jacob from San Jose's primary factor is, "My friends. It is a very close group who go out often and talk often, bonding." Our 911 operator sees kin as the antidote to life's troubles: "There have been times when I have let myself get dragged down into despair … and then I look at my nieces and nephews play and I know I can do better for them."

The single factor that has been emerging in preceding In Their Own Words sections bursts into full view here. Despite the open door of "event, experience or a person," it is a particular person that dominates these responses: one's spouse. Twenty of the fifty qualitative respondents offer statements like the following as singular happiness factors:

My marital experience ... I have someone who supports me 24/7 ...
She (my wife) was married to me for 37 years and she gave me a purpose in life.
When I signed the divorce papers.
My wife. She is a wonderful, brilliant person and that makes things interesting.
My husband. It is good to go through life with a partner you can rely on ... I definitely would get married again.

Again, the point here is not quantification; that is the domain of General Social Survey analyses. But what is apparent in this profusion of heartfelt statements is the core issue of Chap. 7: causality. A plurality of respondents have no trouble identifying their spouses as prime movers of happiness.

In My Own Words

This book has been the destination of a long journey. Over two decades ago, I decided to take stock of American society. A daunting prospect, but many others—mainly talking heads and academics—had already proclaimed that America was in decline.

I took this conclusion to be wildly premature, but the resources were available to find out. Using the General Social Survey, I constructed a model of social capital, defined as the everyday social structures we build and maintain to seek the things we value—specifically: work, family, voluntary association, and social networks. In my last book, *Social Capital in American Life*, I incorporated the attitudes associated with social capital, including job satisfaction, marital happiness and, most to the point, happiness itself.

Now since they are used to "seek the things we value," the theoretical and commonsensical expectation is that the forms of social capital would have some happiness payoff. They did in the last book, and they resoundingly do so in this book.

So: the subtitle A Sociological Perspective is not an exploration, but a declaration. The findings are based on five decades of unimpeachable quantitative data and fifty qualitative interviews of a cross-section of Americans. To this number-crunching researcher, the latter have been both a revelation and a confirmation. Clearly, mixed methods can be synergistic.

This should not be taken as a denial of other perspectives on happiness. Psychological issues such as depression and anxiety have emerged here unbidden. Several respondents even described an existential path of personal development. But to suppose that social relations are not prominent on those paths at this point would seem myopic. Religion is another happiness source for some, but no one would suppose that it does not have sociological features. Cases can be made for multiple perspectives on happiness; the case for sociology is now closed.

NOTES

1. Michael Davern, Rene Bautista, Jeremy Freese, Stephen L. Morgan and Tom. W. Smith, *2016–2020 GSS Panel Codebook*, Release 1a, (National Opinion Research Center, Chicago, 2021).
2. Chi-square = 29.544, $p < 0.001$.
3. Each happiness item is scored 1–3, then the 2018 score is subtracted from the 2020 score to determine the direction of change.
4. Chi-square = 30.531, $p < 0.001$.
5. Mean emails hours per week change = -1.453, mean TV hours per day change = +0.6009.
6. For the main effect of subjective social class, $F = 4.106$, $p = 0.006$.
7. For the main effect of network socializing, $F = 2.011$, $p = 0.134$.
8. For the main effect of marital status, $F = 67.126$, $p < 0.001$.
9. For the main effect of marital status, $F = 22.959$, $p < 0.001$; for the main effect of network socializing, $F = 3.070$, $p = 0.047$.

REFERENCE

Davern, Michael, Rene Bautista, Jeremy Freese, Stephen L. Morgan, and Tom W. Smith, *2016–2020 GSS Panel Codebook*, Release 1a, (National Opinion Research Center, Chicago, 2021).

Index[1]

[1] Note: Page numbers followed by 'n' refer to notes.

© The Author(s), under exclusive license to Springer Nature
Switzerland AG 2024
B. J. Jones, *The Pursuit of Happiness in America*,
https://doi.org/10.1007/978-3-031-65607-1

Printed in the United States
by Baker & Taylor Publisher Services